CRC Desk Reference on
SPORTS NUTRITION

CRC *Desk Reference on*
SPORTS
NUTRITION

MARK KERN, Ph.D., R.D.

Department of Exercise and Nutritional Sciences
San Diego State University
San Diego, California

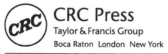

CRC Press
Taylor & Francis Group
Boca Raton London New York

CRC Press is an imprint of the
Taylor & Francis Group, an **informa** business
A TAYLOR & FRANCIS BOOK

Published 2005 by CRC Press
Taylor & Francis Group
6000 Broken Sound Parkway NW, Suite 300
Boca Raton, FL 33487-2742

© 2005 by Taylor & Francis Group, LLC
CRC Press is an imprint of Taylor & Francis Group, an Informa business

First issued in paperback 2019

No claim to original U.S. Government works

ISBN-13: 978-0-367-45415-9 (pbk)
ISBN-13: 978-0-8493-2273-0 (hbk)

Library of Congress Card Number 2004064946

Visit the Taylor & Francis Web site at
http://www.taylorandfrancis.com

and the CRC Press Web site at
http://www.crcpress.com

Library of Congress Cataloging-in-Publication Data

Kern, Mark.
    CRC desk reference on sports nutrition / Mark Kern.
        p. cm.
    Includes bibliographical references.
    ISBN 0-8493-2273-1 (alk. paper)
        1. Athletes—Nutrition. I. Title.

TX361.A8K47 2005
613.2'024'796—dc22   2004064946

Preface

Sports nutrition has become a critical issue in the world of nutrition. This specialty encompasses the assessment of the nutritional status of athletes as well as the effects of exercise, diet, and dietary supplements on metabolism and performance. Athletes, dietitians, and other nutrition practitioners, coaches, and athletic trainers require knowledge of nutrition that can be applied to sports in a manner that can enhance health and performance.

This book provides a collection of alphabetical entries of terms and concepts central to the area of sports nutrition with the goal of providing concise, up-to-date information for the reader. Each entry is provided in one of the following formats: definition—limited to 50 words; paragraph—approximately 51 to 100 words; essay—101 to 300 words; composition—301 to 600 words; article—601 to 1000 words; feature article—1001+ words. Entries were selected based on their relevance to sports nutrition, and depth of coverage was determined by the importance to the field and the volume of available research for review. Collaborating authors with specific knowledge and experiences contributed several entries.

This book can serve as a valuable resource for registered dietitians, sports medicine physicians, athletic trainers, coaches, strength and conditioning coaches, researchers, and others interested in sports nutrition. While intended as a desk reference, it can also be an excellent addition to the holdings of college and high school libraries. Since many terms used in the longer entries have been defined in separate entries, this book can be useful to a wide variety of audiences.

Author

Mark Kern, Ph.D., R.D., received his B.S. and M.S. degrees in nutrition science at Indiana University in Bloomington, Indiana, and his Ph.D. in foods and nutrition at Purdue University. He completed his dietetics training at Ball Memorial Hospital in Muncie, Indiana. Dr. Kern has been a member of the faculty in the Department of Exercise and Nutritional Sciences at San Diego State University since 1995.

Dr. Kern's major research interests include sports dietetics as well as the independent and interactive effects of diet and exercise on risk for chronic diseases. He is an active member of the Sports, Cardiovascular, and Wellness Nutritionists Dietetic Practice Group of the American Dietetic Association and serves as the Editor-in-Chief of *PULSE*, the organization's quarterly peer-reviewed publication. He is also a member of several other professional societies and serves as a reviewer for several peer-reviewed journals.

Contributors

Yael Melamud Pernick, M.S.
San Diego State University
San Diego, California

Amy R. Culp, R.D., L.D.
sCULPture Nutrition & Fitness
Leander, Texas

Natalie Ledesma, M.S., R.D.
Medical Center
University of California, San Francisco
San Francisco, California

Acknowledgments

The author thanks his contributing authors: Yael Pernick, Amy Culp, and Natalie Ledesma. Their friendship and excellent contributions are very much appreciated. I would also like to thank Pat Roberson, Fiona MacDonald, and Susan Farmer of Taylor & Francis for their work on this project. Lastly, I would like Katie and Jenny to know how much I appreciate their support—thanks a bunch!

A

Absorption is the movement of a nutrient or other substance from within the lumen of the gastrointestinal tract to the bloodstream via either the portal circulation or the lymphatic system. In general, water-soluble nutrients are absorbed via the portal circulation and lipid-soluble nutrients are absorbed via the lymphatic system. The primary mechanisms of nutrient absorption are diffusion, facilitated diffusion, and active transport.

For athletes, the rate of absorption of nutrients from foods can be important for optimal athletic performance. For example, foods that produce a delay in absorption of carbohydrates can reduce the rate at which glucose is available to working muscles for energy production and limit exercise capacity. On the other hand, some researchers have suggested a decrease in the rate of glucose absorption in preexercise feedings may actually improve performance by producing a steadier increase in blood glucose and insulin concentrations.

Acclimatization (or acclimation) is an adaptation of the body to an external stress such as heat or altitude. Athletes typically acclimate to high environmental temperatures within a few weeks through enhanced ability to dissipate heat via several mechanisms including blood volume expansion and an increased sweating capacity. These adaptations can result in lower core body temperatures during exercise, which can translate to improved performance. Acclimatization to high altitudes can also result in increased physical work capacity through stimulation of red blood cell production, also termed erythropoiesis.

Acetic acid is a short chain, two-carbon, fatty acid that is integral in metabolism, particularly as a part of acetyl CoA.

Acetyl CoA is composed of acetic acid and coenzyme A and is a vital molecule in intermediary metabolism. It is produced in the catabolism of macronutrients and is required for the synthesis of many important compounds, including fatty acids, cholesterol, and ketones.

Acetylcholine is a neurotransmitter released by nerve endings at the neuromuscular junction in response to an action potential.

Acidosis is a condition of excess acid accumulation and thus a low pH in the body. Typical body pH is approximately 7.4. In sports, transient acidosis occurs when the rate of acid production (e.g., lactic acid, etc.) exceeds the rate of removal.

Actin Along with myosin, actin is one of the two principal contractile proteins in the muscle cell.

Active transport is a process whereby a substance moves from one side of a cell to the other, as in the absorption of several nutrients. This process requires energy from adenosine triphosphate (ATP) and a carrier molecule. Nutrients absorbed via active transport can be absorbed against a concentration gradient.

Additives are substances used in food processing to achieve improved stability, flavor, color, or texture. All additives in the United States' food supply must be generally recognized as safe (GRAS) according to the Food and Drug Administration.

Adenosine triphosphate (ATP) (Figure A.1) is a high-energy phosphate compound required by the majority of energy-requiring processes in the body. The energy produced in the splitting of the high-energy phosphate bond of ATP is approximately 7300 cal/mol. That energy can be used to drive endothermic (energy-requiring) reactions in the body. Processes that require ATP for functioning include muscular contraction, active transport, and many biosynthetic reactions of the body.

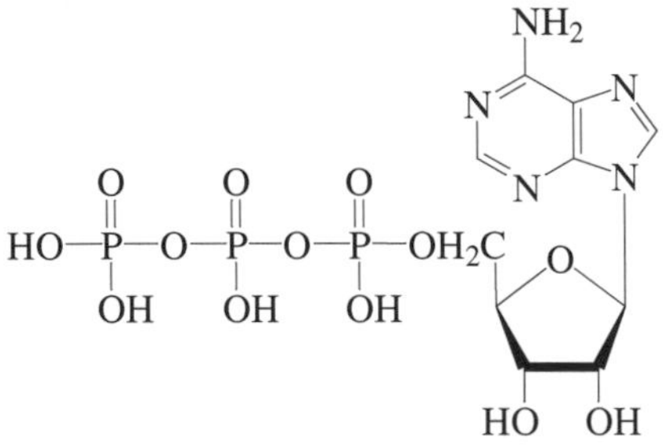

ATP (adenosine triphosphate)

FIGURE A.1

Adequate Intake (AI) The Adequate Intake value is one of four possible Dietary Reference Intake (DRI) values established for a nutrient by the Food and Nutrition Board of the National Academy of Sciences. The AI represents the level of a nutrient that is estimated to meet the needs of most healthy people within a specific age range and gender when there is a lack of data to establish a Recommended Dietary Allowance (RDA) value.

Aerobic exercise The term aerobic is used to refer to reactions or organisms that require oxygen. When applied to exercise, this term is used to describe types of activity in which aerobic metabolism predominates and can be continued for an extended period of time. Examples of aerobic exercise can include various types of "aerobics," such as walking, jogging, running, swimming, cycling, and so forth. Sports can also include a large aerobic component that is often mixed with anaerobic periods of exercise. Team sports such as hockey, basketball, soccer, and many others typically include an aerobic component.

Aerobic glycolysis Glycolysis is a several-step process whereby energy is produced by the breakdown of glucose. When glucose is broken down "aerobically," the endpoint of glycolysis is pyruvic acid, also known as pyruvate. Pyruvate and its products can then continue to produce energy through a series of several metabolic reactions and pathways including the pyruvate dehydrogenase complex, Krebs cycle, and the electron transport system.

AI *See* **Adequate Intake**

Alanine (Figure A.2) is a nonessential amino acid needed for the production of proteins. It is also a highly gluconeogenic amino acid as explained in the entry for the alanine cycle. Interestingly, it is considered the amino acid with the highest rate of oxidation for energy.[1,2] Alanine supplementation has been demonstrated to spare the use of essential amino acids as an energy source under some conditions.[3-5]

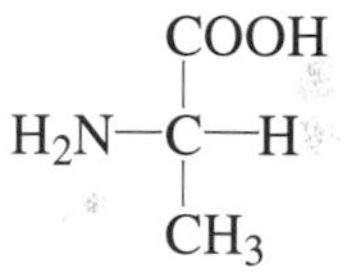

$$\text{COOH}$$
$$|$$
$$\text{H}_2\text{N}-\text{C}-\text{H}$$
$$|$$
$$\text{CH}_3$$

alanine

FIGURE A.2

Little research has been attempted to establish an ergogenic role of alanine. In a recent study, however, the ergogenic potential was examined as was its influence on plasma concentrations of amino acids and fuel substrates.[6] In a double blind design, four different solutions containing 6% of alanine and 6% of sucrose (ALA-CHO); 6% of ALA; 6% of CHO; and a placebo (PLC) were tested during four trials performed in random order. Ten trained athletes cycled for 45 minutes at 75% of their VO_{2max} followed by a 15-minute performance test. Blood samples were collected prior to the start of exercise and immediately before the 15-minute performance ride. Alanine supplementation with or without sucrose blunted the exercise-induced decrease in plasma concentrations of most other gluconeogenic amino acids but failed to enhance endurance performance.

Alanine cycle is a series of reactions in which alanine obtained in the muscle from pyruvate through a transamination (pyruvate accepts an amino group from a different amino acid) reaction enters the bloodstream and is taken up by the liver for conversion to glucose by gluconeogenesis. Glucose can be secreted from the liver and then taken up by the muscle where it again produces pyruvate through glycolysis, which is now available once again for transamination to alanine.

Alcohol Many chemicals are considered alcohols. The alcohol that is used for human consumption is ethanol, which is derived through the fermentation of carbohydrates. Ethanol provides approximately 7 kcal/g when consumed at low to moderate levels. During excess consumption less energy is produced, because the metabolic system (microsomal ethanol oxidizing system) used in the production of energy from alcohol during times of excess produces less energy.

Ethanol has been used by some athletes as a potential ergogenic aid for many years. While alcoholic beverages contain significant amounts of water, the diuretic effect of alcohol will prevent much of the potential hydrating effect of the water; thus, alcoholic beverages are a poor choice for fluid replacement. Alcoholic beverages also provide energy that can be used as a fuel. When used in limited amounts, alcoholic beverages are not likely to provide adequate fuel to improve exercise performance. At levels providing a significant amount of energy, alcohol is likely to be ergolytic (i.e., performance impairing), however, due to adverse changes in metabolism (for example, hypoglycemia, glycogen depletion, etc.) and the intoxicating effects that often accompany consumption of alcoholic beverages.

As part of the general diet of a nonalcoholic athlete, modest consumption of alcoholic beverages may exert the same currently recognized positive benefits that have been recognized for the general population. Research suggests that alcohol may reduce the risk of cardiovascular disease.[7] Potential mechanisms for this effect include increased concentration of high density lipoprotein cholesterol in the blood, decreased platelet aggregation, and improved antioxidant status.

Amino acids (often referred to as the building blocks of proteins) are characterized by having an amino group, a carboxylic acid group, and a characteristic side chain or residue (R), each bound to a central carbon. The general structure of an amino acid is depicted in Figure A.3. Twenty amino acids are required for the production of the body's proteins, while a few others are not. Most amino acids also have important nonprotein functions. Nine amino acids are considered essential, since they must be supplied by the diet, while the remaining amino acids are nonessential (see Table A.1). Functions and ergogenic effects are provided in separate entries for each amino acid. The entry for protein also

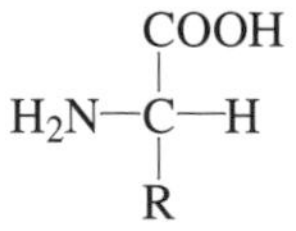

$$
\begin{array}{c}
\text{COOH} \\
| \\
\text{H}_2\text{N}-\text{C}-\text{H} \\
| \\
\text{R}
\end{array}
$$

amino acids
(basic structure)

FIGURE A.3

TABLE A.1
Amino Acids Found in the Diet and the Body

Amino Acids Needed for Protein Structure		Amino Acids that Do Not Form Proteins
Essential Amino Acids	Nonessential Amino Acids	
Phenylalanine	Glycine	Citrulline
Leucine	Alanine	Ornithine
Isoleucine	Serine	Taurine
Valine	Tyrosine	
Histidine	Glutamine	
Lysine	Glutamic acid	
Threonine	Arginine	
Tryptophan	Asparagine	
Methionine	Aspartic acid	
	Threonine	
	Cysteine	

describes some research on the efficacy of amino acid consumption on the development of skeletal muscle.

Anaerobic exercise The term anaerobic is used to refer to reactions or organisms that require no oxygen. When applied to exercise, this term is used to describe types of activity that can only be continued for a short period of time. Oxygen is required by the body during anaerobic exercise; however, a greater percent of the body's energy is provided by anaerobic reactions during this type of activity. Examples of anaerobic exercise can include weight lifting, sprinting, and so forth. Sports requiring high bursts of energy that cannot be sustained for long periods of time also include an important anaerobic component.

Anaerobic glycolysis Glycolysis is a several-step process whereby energy is produced by the breakdown of glucose. When glucose is down "anaerobically," the endpoint of glycolysis is lactic acid, also known as lactate. Lactate is obtained by an anaerobic reaction catalyzed by lactic acid dehydrogenase, which converts pyruvate to lactate. Lactate that is produced in the muscle can diffuse into the bloodstream. This process has been implicated in the eventual production of fatigue, either by the drop in pH or by the lactate molecules directly. When exercise intensity decreases, the lactate can be converted back to glucose via gluconeogenesis. Refer to the entry for glycolysis for more information, including a diagram.

Androstenedione is an intermediate molecule in the synthesis of testosterone from cholesterol. As such, it has received a great deal of attention as a dietary supplementation for athletes, who often refer to it as "andro." Many androstene-related metabolites have been used in a variety of supplemental preparations.

In a study published as an abstract, a mixture of 4-androsten-3, 17 diol; 4-androstene-3, 17-dione; 5-androstene-3, 17-dione; 5-androstene-3, 17-diol; 19-nor-4-androstene-3-17-dione; and 19-nor-5-androstene-3, 17-diol was administered at a dose of 150 mg three times each day for a duration of 4 weeks.[8] No changes in serum concentrations of testosterone, estradiol, or leutinizing hormone were detected; however, the results from this study indicate that the participants gained 2.3% of their body weight and 1.1% of their lean body mass on average. Additionally, the average vertical jump height increased by 9.3% in these participants.

Another study in which 300 mg of androstenedione or a placebo were provided each day during an 8-week resistance training program indicated that plasma estradiol concentration was elevated after 2, 5, and 8 weeks of supplementation.[9] The muscle fiber cross-sectional area and strength as measured by knee extension improved equally between the two groups as did lean body mass. This study suggests that there are no benefits of "andro" supplementation. Furthermore, these researchers determined that plasma concentrations of high-density lipoprotein cholesterol were decreased in androstenedione by approximately 12%, which suggests that long-term "andro" consumption may increase the risk for premature cardiovascular disease in users.

Overall, most research has failed to demonstrate positive changes,[10–12] but it appears that doses of at least 200 to 300 mg per day are required to produce positive changes in testosterone, if at all.[13,14] These changes have not been consistently demonstrated and subsequent positive changes in anabolism or strength have been elusive. Furthermore, doses at or above this level may someday prove to increase the risk for chronic degenerative diseases.

Anion is an ion with a negative charge. The term ion refers to a chemical that has either a positive or negative charge.

Anorexia nervosa *See* **Eating disorders**

Antioxidants are molecules that have the property of neutralizing free radicals and reactive oxygen species (ROS) that are continuously produced as part of metabolic processes. While some of the body's antioxidant defenses are achieved through enzymatic defense systems such as glutathione peroxidase, superoxide dismutase, and catalase, other molecules such as vitamin C, vitamin E, beta-carotene, and many other phytochemicals assist in the body's elaborate defense system.

Intense aerobic and resistance exercises have been shown to increase the production of ROS and free radicals.[15–17] This increase in the generation of free radicals from physical activity occurs in several ways. As oxidative phosphorylation increases in response to exercise, there is a resulting increase in free radicals since 2 to 5% of oxygen used in the mitochondria forms free radicals.[18] Free radicals are also produced by catecholamines in response to exercise. In addition, other sources can contribute to the release of free radicals during exercise, such as prostanoid metabolism, xanthine oxidase, NADPH oxidase, and secondary sources, including the release of radicals by macrophages recruited to repair damaged tissue.[18] There are three mechanisms of free radical production that are of special concern to athletes. These include 1) accelerated metabolic (mostly mitochondrial) oxygen processing; 2) ischemic-reperfusion injury; and 3) muscle microtrauma and repair.[19] Endurance training is mostly associated with accelerated mitochondrial oxygen processing, whereas resistance training is associated with ischemic-reperfusion injury and muscle trauma and repair.[19]

In general, while a bout of exercise can promote oxidative stress, exercise training may produce adaptations that may limit the damage caused by exercise. A review by Powers et al.[15] suggests that the activities of key antioxidant enzymes such as glutathione peroxidase and superoxide dismutase are elevated in exercisers and that training can enhance muscle glutathione status. While many studies support these findings, not all are in agreement.[20] However, as reviewed by Urso and Clarkson,[18] research examining the impact of exercise training on the status of antioxidant enzymes has provided positive evidence of increased activity through studies a) assessing active vs. inactive individuals; b) determining the relationship between training volume and antioxidant status; and c) monitoring changes that occur when less active subjects complete a training program. Overall, these data provide a compelling case to suggest that antioxidant status increases as a natural effect of exercise training.

If free radicals increase to a level greater than the body's ability to neutralize them, the radicals will attack cellular components, especially lipids. An attack on lipids initiates lipid peroxidation, which leads to the generation of more free radicals and ROS that can harm other cellular components such as protein and DNA.[18] The body appears to withstand a limited increase in free radicals, and data suggests that an increase in ROS is necessary for muscle adaptation to occur.

Research does not support an ergogenic effect of antioxidant supplementation, meaning that supplementation does not apparently improve athletic performance. The key issue regarding antioxidants in sports nutrition is the role of dietary or supplemental antioxidants in the protection against oxidative stress encountered under conditions of exercise or training, although it is currently unclear whether strenuous exercise increases this need.[21]

Many studies have examined the effects of antioxidant supplements and have used exercise performance and changes in oxidative stress as measures of outcome. Vitamin C has been widely studied and a review of early studies reveals conflicting results of the use of supplementation on work capacity and anaerobic performance.[22–25] Buzina and Suboticanec indicated that vitamin C was related to aerobic capacity; however, the association was strongest in subjects whose plasma vitamin C levels were initially low.[26] These results suggest that exercise performance may only be enhanced by vitamin C supplementation if there is a deficiency in individuals. However, another study revealed no decrement in aerobic power when vitamin C intake was restricted for 7 weeks.[27]

Additional research has focused on the effects of vitamin C supplementation on countering exercise-induced muscle damage and the reduction of muscle soreness. A study by Kaminski and Boal indicated that 3 days of 3000 g/day of vitamin C supplementation prior to exercise and 4 days after exercise, resulted in less delayed onset of muscle soreness compared to a placebo.[28] However, Thompson and colleagues revealed that plasma vitamin C was increased with one dose of 1000 mg of vitamin C given 2 hours prior to a 90-minute shuttle run, but the development of muscle soreness after the race was not altered.[29] Jakeman and Maxwell reported that subjects recovered strength and contractile function faster after a muscle damaging exercise when supplemented with 400 mg of vitamin C for 21 days compared to subjects taking 400 mg of vitamin E or a placebo.[30] It was thus suggested by the authors that vitamin C may protect cell structures from oxidative stress and free radical damage.

Vitamin E is also a powerful antioxidant and may protect muscles in a fashion similar to vitamin C. No studies have detected an ergogenic effect of vitamin E and most studies do not support vitamin E as a supplement capable of altering metabolism to a degree that could alter performance.[31–35] In addition, Helgheim and colleagues concluded that vitamin E did not alter muscle disruption from exercise.[36] However, a more recent study indicated that 4 weeks of 1200 IU/day of vitamin E reduced the leakage of muscle enzymes in response to a more stressful exercise challenge.[37] Overall, a review of present studies has found that the effect of vitamin E supplementation on the inflammatory response to exercise is unclear.[18]

Another important antioxidant nutrient is beta-carotene, which can also serve as a precursor to vitamin A. Although research does not support an ergogenic effect of beta-carotene, some studies have suggested that its supplementation may confer protection against oxidative stress. In research where the investigators provided a supplemental combination of vitamin C, E, and beta-carotene, decreased levels of lipid peroxidation at rest and during exercise at different intensities were detected.[38] Additionally, a different study reported that this combination of antioxidants has a protective effect on both blood glutathione and muscle damage.[39] It is not possible to determine from this type of research if the antioxidants had separate effects or if the combination was required to induce protection.

Many other nutrients and phytochemicals have been evaluated for their potential roles in reducing exercise-induced oxidative stress. In general, while less research is available for other antioxidants, neither selenium nor CoQ_{10}, appear to enhance performance or prevent accumulation of free radical species and oxidation. However, selenium supplementation has been demonstrated to improve glutathione status in some limited research.[40] Research generally does not support a potential capacity for CoQ_{10} to reduce oxidative stress. In fact, some researchers have detected adverse effects[41] and even decreased performance.[41,42]

In conclusion, research does not currently support the necessity of antioxidant supplementation for athletes to enhance performance, although some research does suggest that supplementation may decrease the oxidative stress of exercise. Interestingly, protection against exercise-induced oxidative stress appears to occur naturally with exercise training. Overall, the most prudent recommendation to date is for an athlete to consume a diet naturally rich in antioxidants.

Appetite During weight balance, food intake and energy expenditure are closely linked and individuals, such as athletes, who expend a large amount of energy will require consumption of an equal amount of energy and those expending low amounts of energy will require a lower energy intake. Interestingly, however, for those initiating an exercise program, research suggests that energy intake and expenditure are not quite so tightly linked and energy intake may not match energy expenditure, leading to weight loss. One explanation is that the appetite may be suppressed, perhaps due to elevated core body temperature, following a vigorous bout of exercise. Although exercise may play a role in determining appetite, many other factors aside from exercise have strong influences on food intake.

Arginine (Figure A.4) is a dibasic, nonessential amino acid. Oral arginine supplements are often marketed as enhancers of human growth hormone, which appears to exert its anabolic effects through insulin-like growth factor-1 (IFG-1). Interestingly, research does not support a role of elevations in growth hormone with increases in lean body mass or strength in individuals with previously normal levels of growth hormone. Additionally, most well-controlled studies do not support a role for oral arginine supplementation in enhancing growth hormone concentrations. Although a few studies have detected an increase in concentration of growth hormone, they have not successfully linked this shift to enhanced lean body mass or strength. In many studies, arginine has been fed in combination with other amino acids including lysine, ornithine, and glutamate with similar results to supplementation with arginine alone. In some cases, studies have attempted to determine if arginine alone or in combination with other amino acids can enhance the typical elevation in growth hormone observed with a bout of exercise. The results of these studies have not supported a growth hormone-enhancing effect.[43]

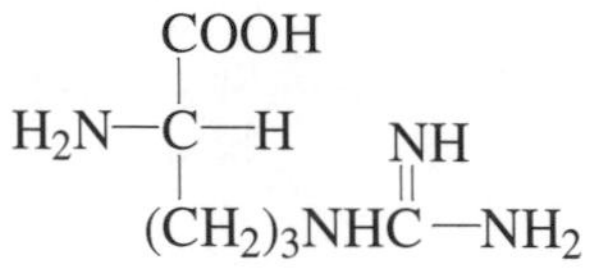

$$COOH$$
$$H_2N-C-H$$
$$(CH_2)_3NHC-NH \quad (NH)$$

arginine

FIGURE A.4

Arsenic is a micromineral most often thought of as a potentially lethal substance. Within the diet, arsenic is particularly rich in seafood, but is also found in trace quantities in grains, vegetables, fruits, dairy foods, meat, and eggs. The essentiality of arsenic has been an area of controversy, but it appears to have a role in the metabolism of amino acids such as methionine and arginine.

Ascorbic acid *See* **Vitamin C**

Asparagine (Figure A.5) is a nonessential amino acid. It is an integral component of the body's proteins and serves as a major donor of amine groups for the production of other compounds.

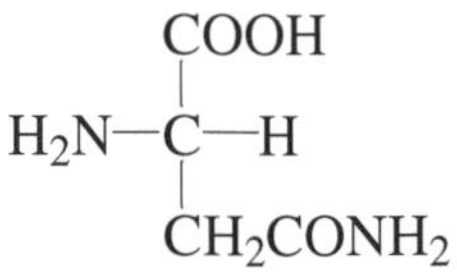

$$COOH$$
$$H_2N-C-H$$
$$CH_2CONH_2$$

asparagine

FIGURE A.5

Aspartic acid (see Figure A.6), also referred to as aspartate, is a nonessential amino acid required for the synthesis of proteins. It is also required for the production of purines and pyrimidines and is essential for the elimination of nitrogen from the body through the production of urea.

Salts of aspartate, particularly potassium and magnesium, have been used as ergogenic aids for many years. Although not all research is in agreement, several studies have suggested that supplements of aspartate salts may decrease ammonia accumulation and enhance endurance performance.[44–46] Others studies have failed to detect similar effects.[47–49] Less research has examined the potential for aspartate salts to improve strength, but most studies have failed to detect increased strength or decreased plasma ammonia concentration during and after resistance training.[50,51]

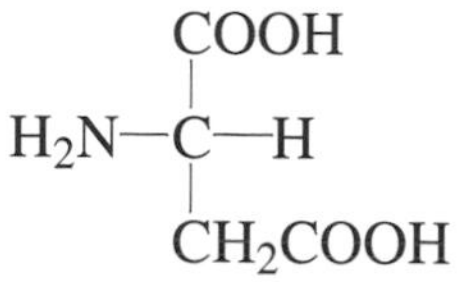

$$COOH$$
$$H_2N-C-H$$
$$CH_2COOH$$

aspartic acid

FIGURE A.6

Atherosclerosis is the formation of plaque along the walls of blood vessels, which causes "hardening of the arteries." As the opening of the blood vessel narrows due to plaque accumulation, risk for loss of blood supply to that part of the body occurs. Many nutritional and nonnutritional factors are responsible for the formation of these plaques. Exercise is important for the prevention of atherosclerosis.

Athlete An athlete is a person who competes in a sporting event. Athletes who are extremely well trained for their particular sports are often referred to as elite athletes.

Atwater factors The values used to express the amount of energy that is available from a gram of any macronutrient are often termed Atwater factors, after the researcher most credited for their determination, W. O. Atwater. Fat, protein, carbohydrate, and alcohol are typically estimated to provide 9, 4, 4, and 7 kcal/g, respectively.

B

Baking soda *See* **Sodium bicarbonate**

Basal metabolic rate (BMR) The level of energy expended at rest following an overnight fast is considered the basal metabolic rate (BMR). Thus, BMR describes the lowest amount of energy that must be expended to support the body's physiological processes. This differs from resting metabolic rate (RMR), also known as resting energy expenditure, only RMR is not always measured following an overnight fast prior to any of the days' activities. Body weight accounts for approximately 75% of variation among individuals' BMR, with the level lean body mass being the most important component.[52] Vital organs, such as the brain, liver, heart, and kidneys expend much of the basal energy. Interestingly, active transport processes (the movement of particles across cellular membranes that requires energy) contribute significantly to BMR.

The BMR of physically trained individuals has been studied extensively to determine if it may partially account for the lower rates of overweight and obesity in this population. While some studies have suggested that training increases BMR, other studies have not supported this notion.[53] Since lean body mass accounts for much of the BMR, an individual who increases his or her musculature during training is likely to have a higher BMR. However, in general it seems that basal energy expenditure is not altered by exercise training when body composition is unchanged. Exercisers who lose weight are likely to experience a decrease in BMR. This is particularly true when weight loss is rapid and a portion of the weight loss is lean tissue. To prevent a loss in lean body mass during weight loss, the rate of weight loss must be gradual and exercise should include some resistance training.

BCAA *See* **Branched-chain amino acids**

Bee pollen has been marketed as a dietary supplement and used by athletes for many years. While bee pollen contains many essential nutrients (such as protein, vitamins, and minerals), its ability to improve athletic performance is unlikely in a well-nourished athlete. Well-designed studies have failed to provide any evidence that bee pollen can promote enhanced physical performance.[54] Furthermore, there is some risk of an allergic reaction to its consumption.

B

Beriberi The deficiency syndrome of thiamin (vitamin B_1) is known as beriberi, which can have three different forms and include muscular weakness and wasting as well as cardiovascular abnormalities. While physical activity will increase the demands for energy intake and thus thiamin, it is not likely that an athlete will suffer from beriberi.

Beta-carotene is among a group of pigments known as carotenoids and is a major source and precursor of vitamin A.[55,56] Carotenes are colored pigments found in yellow and green vegetables. Many carotenes, including beta-carotene, are chain-breaking antioxidants and singlet oxygen quenchers. Thus, beta-carotene functions as one of the many antioxidants in the human body[56] that are considered to inhibit the oxidative modification of low-density lipoproteins, inhibiting the atherosclerotic process and the subsequent progression of coronary heart disease.[57] However, the belief that antioxidant supplements can prevent heart disease has not been proven by clinical evidence.[58–60]

Most studies have shown that supplementation of beta-carotene typically neither causes harm nor offers benefit for disease risk; therefore, beta-carotene supplementation does not seem to improve oxidative status and needs are likely met by the diet in most individuals.[55] Muscular exercise results in an increased production of free radicals. Although some animal experiments have confirmed that adding antioxidants to the diet can improve muscular repair and perhaps performance, to date there is serious lack of evidence showing that supplementing with antioxidants actually improves human performance.[61]

Beta-hydroxy-beta-methylbutyrate (HMB) has been available as a dietary supplement for several years. HMB is produced during the metabolism of leucine, but is not considered an essential nutrient itself. Initial research suggested that in untrained subjects who initiated a 3-week resistance training program, daily supplementation of 1.5 and 3.0 daily grams of HMB exhibited enhanced strength and lean body mass in comparison to resistance training only.[62]

The potential mechanism for improvement that was suggested by those researchers was decreased muscle catabolism, since urinary excretion of 3-methylhistidine was lower in the HMB-supplemented groups. If HMB is truly capable of preventing muscle breakdown, supplementation during resistance exercise could theoretically enhance net positive changes in lean mass. The efficacy of HMB may depend on the state of training, however, since later research in already trained individuals (as well as a longer follow-up of subjects who gained lean body mass and strength after 3 weeks of supplementation and training) failed to detect further gains in lean mass and strength.

Beta-oxidation is the metabolic process in which fatty acids in the mitochondria are oxidized, producing acetyl CoA, NADH + H$^+$, and FADH$_2$.

Beverages *See* **Sports drinks**

BIA *See* **Bioelectrical impedance analysis**

Bicarbonate *See* **Sodium bicarbonate**

Bile is a fluid containing bile acids that are synthesized in the liver. Bile is stored and concentrated in the gallbladder from which it is released in response to a meal to allow for digestion and subsequent absorption of fat.

Bile acids are synthesized from cholesterol in the liver. At physiological pH levels, bile acids are present as anions and are referred to as bile salts. The primary functions of bile acids are to aid in the digestion and absorption of fats.

Bioavailability The amount of a nutrient utilized from the diet for function within the body is used to describe the nutrient's bioavailability.

Bioelectrical impedance analysis (BIA) is a method for determining body composition. The determination of body fat is performed by passing a harmless electrical current through the body. The conductance is detected as the resistance of the body mass to the electrical current. The resistance is greatest in fat tissue, which has only 14 to 22% water, and the conductance is greatest in fat-free tissue.[63] Through electrical conductance, a BIA meter can determine the total body water content and use various formulas to calculate lean body mass and fat mass after taking body mass, stature, sex, age, and sometimes race into consideration.[63,64] When comparing the BIA to other methods of body composition, such as the hydrodensitometry and skinfold calipers, Pearson correlations for male and female body fat percentages were found to be high between the three methods, ranging from 0.81 to 0.86.[65]

There has been substantial attention in the fields of sports and exercise on the use of BIA in the evaluation of body composition because body composition has a significant effect on athletic performance and because exercise has the potential to modify body composition. Body composition is an important determinant of performance in many sports. Consequently, there is a need for a body-composition assessment technique that is safe, noninvasive, rapid, reliable, accurate, and sensitive to the small differences in body composition that may take place during training. BIA apparently meets many of these needs: measurements are performed rapidly and noninvasively, the method is relatively inexpensive, and when used under proper testing conditions it is appropriate for comparative character-ization of the body composition of athletes in different sports.[66]

However, there are several potential confounding problems with the use of BIA in athletes, for example, hydration, skin temperature, the last bout of exercise, glycogen stores, and chemical maturity in younger athletes. Previous diet and exercise are also important factors in the use of impedance in athletes before competition. For instance, carbohydrate-loading tends to raise estimated fat-free mass (FFM) because of the extra water bound to glycogen. In addition, exercise can affect measured body resistance by increasing vascular perfusion, hyperemia, cutaneous blood flow, and vasodilation. Therefore, it is recommended to wait several hours after strenuous exercise before impedance measurements are made.

Biotin (Figure B.1) is a water-soluble vita-min within the B-complex. The pri-mary function of biotin is to act as a cofactor in carboxylation reac-tions. Key processes that require biotin include the conversion of pyruvate to oxalocetate and malonyl CoA synthesis from acetyl CoA for fatty acid synthesis. Deficiency symptoms for biotin include muscle

biotin

FIGURE B.1

pain, hallucinations, depression, and nausea. While deficiency of biotin is likely to impair athletic ability, research does not indicate that biotin supplementation in a well-nourished athlete will improve performance. Although studies of supplementation of only biotin on athletic performance are not available, studies in which biotin was included as part of a multivitamin supplement have not demonstrated improvements.[67,68]

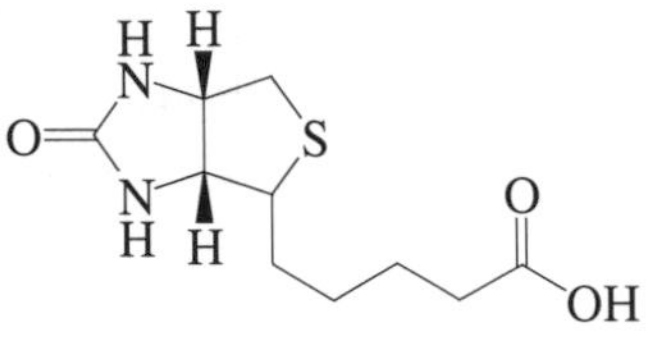

Blood glucose Glucose is a six-carbon sugar, which mainly appears in the body as a result of the ingestion of dietary sources containing carbo-hydrates. Normal blood glucose is approximately 70 to 110 mg/dl, which is the level required for normal function of the central nervous system and other organs and cells. Blood glucose below normal con-centrations is referred to as hypoglycemia, while blood glucose greater than normal is hyperglycemia. During rest, glucose enters the cells via the action of glucose transporters. The GLUT-4 transporter appears to be primarily responsible and activated by the hormone insulin. During exercise, insulin levels decline, which suggests that either increased insulin sensitivity is occurring or that glucose is taken up by other mechanisms as well. Since the demand for glucose by the muscles increases during exercise, glucose is released from the liver in the circulation to allow for uptake by the tissues and for the production of energy.[69]

During intense exercise, blood glucose utilization increases sharply with time and can supply up to 30% of the total energy required with muscular glycogen supplying most of the remaining energy requirements.[70] During prolonged exercise, blood glucose becomes a major contributor as muscle glycogen availability is diminished. Once the liver's output of glucose fails to sustain the muscle's glucose uptake, blood glucose levels decrease significantly and might even fall to hypoglycemic values. When carbohydrate stores are depleted, work capacity decreases as well.[70]

Blood pressure is the pressure exerted by blood against the walls of the blood vessels. Systolic blood pressure is the blood pressure during the contraction of the heart, while diastolic blood pressure is the pressure during the relaxation phase of the heart. When a person has high blood pressure, he or she is considered to have hypertension. Conversely, low blood pressure is referred to as hypotension. See the hypertension entry for a brief discussion on the role of exercise in its prevention.

BMD *See* **Bone mineral density**

BMI *See* **Body mass index**

BMR *See* **Basal metabolic rate**

Bodybuilders The dietary goals of bodybuilders are often different from those of endurance or team athletes. For example, the key goal for a bodybuilder is typically to enhance the development of lean body mass and to prevent the accumulation of excess body fat for the purpose of aesthetics rather than athletic performance. While many of the principles regarding nutrition for strength, lean body mass development, and energy production for workouts apply similarly to bodybuilders and other strength-training athletes, research regarding the strategies used by bodybuilders for competition is sorely lacking. Current dietary practices for bodybuilding near the time of competition can be very extreme. These athletes should avoid engaging in any practice that can put their health at risk for either acute or chronic conditions.

Body composition can have a major impact on athletic performance. In some cases a high degree of muscularity (such as bodybuilding, weight lifting, football, and so forth) is essential for optimal performance, while in others (for example, running, etc.) excess muscularity could be a physical hindrance to performance. Similarly, excess body fatness can decrease performance in many sports, yet body fat can be

B

used to the advantage of some athletes (including sumo wrestlers, football lineman, and so on). Determining the optimal level of musculature or fatness for an individual athlete is wrought with problems. For example, not all athletes will perform equally well with identical body compositions. Furthermore, accurate assessment of body composition can be difficult; thus, striving to achieve a particular body fat is not always effective.

Many techniques for assessment of body composition are available. Of those that are used most commonly in research settings, hydrostatic weighing and dual energy x-ray absorptiometry are often considered the most accurate. Other common techniques include calculations based on various body circumferences, skinfold measurements, and bioelectrical impedance analysis, which is now widely available in exercise facilities as well as for home use.

Body fat Assessment of body composition typically involves compartmentalizing the body into either lean body mass or body fat, which is usually expressed as a percentage. For each individual, a certain amount of fat is essential for normal body function. Above that level, body fatness may influence athletic performance in either positive or negative ways as described in the entry on body composition.

Body mass index (BMI) Many indexes of body mass have been developed. The index most commonly used is Quetelet's Index, which is calculated as the weight of an individual in kilograms divided by the square of their height in meters. Body mass index is thus an expression of weight for height and can be useful in determining risk for chronic diseases in which obesity is a risk factor. Since BMI does not always provide an indication of body composition, however, it is not always an adequate predictor of disease risk for individuals.

Bone mineral density (BMD) Bone is a dynamic tissue matrix of collagen and minerals, which consists of 75% water. Bone tissue also contains crystalline salts that are composed of calcium and phosphorous, but which also include a variety of other minerals. There are two primary types of bone cells, also known as osteocytes. Osteoblasts build bone by the process of calcification, while osteoclasts cause the breakdown of bone by the process of mineral resorption. From birth to death, bone tissue is continually being formed, broken down, and reformed in a process called remodeling. During bone maintenance, osteoblastic and osteoclastic activities are in balance. During periods of growth, the activity of osteoblasts exceeds that of osteoclasts until peak bone mineral density is achieved, which is typically observed between the ages of 18 to 25 years in women,[71] although recent research has suggested BMD may peak even sooner in some bone sites.[72] Later in adulthood, osteoclastic activity exceeds osteoblastic activity, resulting in a gradual loss of bone mass, which occurs in women at a much faster rate following menopause.[69]

When bone mineral loss becomes severe, osteopenia and osteoporosis can develop. Osteopenia is often considered a milder condition than osteoporosis, yet is characterized similarly by a low BMD. Eventually the bones progressively become porous and brittle. Osteoporosis is a condition in which even a small trauma can lead to fractures, most commonly in the hip, wrist, or spine.[69] Osteoporosis affects 25 million individuals in the U.S. and causes 1.5 million fractures each year.[73]

The overall impression of the relationship between athletic activity and BMD is that a moderate amount of exercise has a positive impact on bone. One consistent finding in the literature is that moderate physical activity of a weight-bearing nature, such as running or jumping, generally has a more positive impact on bone than nonweight-bearing activities, such as swimming, which along with other activities provide only minimal bone loading appear to have little or no impact on bone.[74] The ideal exercises to enhance BMD seem to involve high-impact activities and progressive resistance training using several slow repetitions at 70 to 80% of the one repetition maximum.[75]

Conversely, some young athletes might suffer from loss of BMD.[76] The prevalence of amenorrhea among female athletes due to low estrogen production often secondary to inadequate energy intake to meet the energy expenditure of an athlete ranges between 3.4 to 66.0%, depending on the population studied.[77] BMD is inversely related to the duration of amenorrhea and the severity of estrogen deficiency.[74] When female athletes experience bone loss due to inadequate estrogen production associated with eating disorders, they are experiencing what has been called the female athlete triad, which is described more completely in a separate entry.

Boron is considered a trace mineral and although relatively little is known about it in comparison to many other minerals, some researchers have suggested that it may be an essential nutrient. Primary dietary sources include some fruits, leafy vegetables, nuts, legumes, and dairy foods. Since much of the boron in the body is found within the bone, a potential role of boron appears to be in production and function of normal bone tissue. Some researchers have also speculated that boron is important for steroid hormone production, which may be the reason for its role in bone health.

When boron deficiency was induced by a diet low in boron, subsequent boron supplementation produced higher plasma concentra-

B

tions of testosterone and reduced urinary calcium and magnesium excretion.[78] This research led to a vast marketing of boron as an ergogenic aid capable of producing steroid-like effects for bodybuilders and weight trainers. However, that study merely suggests that adequate boron is important for normal steroid hormone levels and bone-related mineral balance. Research of boron supplementation in adequately nourished individuals has failed to produce similar results.[79] Furthermore, research on boron supplementation has indicated that boron does not increase lean body mass or strength in bodybuilders. Overall, much is yet to be learned about boron metabolism, but research conducted to date does not support its use as an ergogenic aid for well-nourished athletes.

Bowel The term bowel is used to refer to the intestinal tract. Specifically, most individuals use the word bowel when discussing the large intestine.

Branched-chain amino acids (BCAA) are those amino acids with a branch in their hydrocarbon side-chain. These amino acids include leucine, isoleucine, and valine. BCAA are often described separately from other amino acids not only because of their similarities in structure, but also their similarities in function. In particular, unlike other amino acids, BCAA (especially leucine) can be oxidized to some extent for energy in nonhepatic tissues, such as the muscle, which is one reason that BCAA have received much attention as potential ergogenic aids.

Since BCAA can be used, at least to some extent, directly by muscle cells for energy, supplementation has been theorized to improve endurance exercise performance by providing the muscles with an alternative energy source. Others have theorized that when BCAA are used extensively by muscle tissue for energy during exercise, their concentration in the plasma drops. Simultaneously, free fatty acid bound tryptophan is liberated during the catabolism of the fatty acids for energy. When this occurs, the ratio of BCAA to tryptophan in the plasma decreases, which produces an increased uptake of tryptophan by the brain. When tryptophan enters the brain, serotonin production increases, which may produce the sensation of fatigue. This typically occurs to the greatest extent late in endurance exercise as stores of glycogen are diminished and a reliance on BCAA and free fatty acids for energy increases.[80] This process has been referred to as the central fatigue theory and is described in a separate entry.

Many studies have been conducted to determine if BCAA supplementation, either as separate BCAA or in various combinations, can enhance endurance exercise performance. Separate entries for leucine, isoleucine, and valine are also provided.

Since BCAA supplementation is theorized to improve performance by providing energy to working muscles or to prevent an exercise-induced decrease in plasma concentrations of BCAA, BCAA supplements have been primarily studied using acute feedings prior to or during exercise. In one study, an 18-g mixture of BCAA was added to 175 g of carbohydrate dissolved in a 5% solution and compared to a solution containing the carbohydrate only and a placebo beverage during a 100 km cycling time trial.[81] No differences in performance were detected among the trials. However, in a study performed under conditions of high ambient temperature (~34°C), branched-chain amino acid supplementation significantly improved endurance.[82] In that study, men and women consumed 5 ml of a drink per kg body weight that contained either 5.88 g/l of branched-chain amino acids (19% isoleucine, 27% valine, 54% leucine) or a placebo before and during exercise. Performance in the heat was improved by BCAA supplementation relative to placebo. Whether similar results would have been obtained in cooler conditions is uncertain.

Other studies have also detected either increases in performance or improvements in subjective measures of fatigue. In an early study, marathon running times were improved by prerace BCAA supplementation for "slower" runners but not "faster" runners.[83] In some research, BCAA administration also appears to preserve muscle glycogen.[84]

Most research, however, has failed to provide evidence that BCAA supplementation improves exercise performance. In another study, 7 g/L of branched-chain amino acids were provided along with a carbohydrate beverage in one trial, while the carbohydrate beverage alone was provided in the other.[85] No difference in endurance was detected between the two trials. Similar results were detected in yet another study employing a similar design, but including groups consuming BCAA at two different doses (6 g/L or 18 g/L).[86] In that study neither dose produced improvements in endurance performance.

Overall, the preponderance of research of BCAA supplementation suggests that they are not effective in enhancing endurance performance. Nevertheless, some studies have reported an ergogenic effect of BCAA supplementation and many studies support the notion that a drop in plasma concentrations of BCAA can lead to increased serotonin production. Furthermore, unless the central fatigue theory is disproved, it remains possible that BCAA supplementation may help to prevent fatigue under certain circumstances.

B

Buffer An acid-base buffer is a chemical substance or solution that produces resistance to change in pH. During exercise, metabolism is directed toward the production of an acidic environment. Many nutrients and supplements have been marketed for the potential to produce a buffering capacity, thereby having an ergogenic effect. Most commonly, these substances, such as sodium bicarbonate, are used to enhance performance of relatively short, very intense bouts of exercise. While in some cases buffering aids have been demonstrated to be effective, other compounds used to buffer acid production have been less successful.

Bulimia nervosa *See* **Eating disorders**

B-vitamins (often referred to as the B-complex of vitamins) currently include thiamin (B-1), riboflavin (B-2), niacin (formerly known as B-3), pantothenic acid (formerly known as B-5), pyridoxine and related molecules (B-6), cobalamins (B-12), folic acid (folate, folacin), and biotin. Along with vitamin C (ascorbic acid), these vitamins are classified as the water-soluble vitamins. While many of the B-vitamins have some related functions (such as red blood cell synthesis, energy production from macronutrients, and so forth) and often even interact in metabolism, they each have distinctly different structures and characteristics. Separate entries are provided for each B-vitamin as well as choline. These entries describe the functions, food sources, and ergogenic potential of each vitamin.

C

Caffeine belongs to a group of lipid-soluble compounds called methylxan-
thines. Together, caffeine and related substances such as theophylline
and theobromine are naturally found in coffee beans, tea leaves, choc-
olate, cocoa beans, and cola nuts. Depending on the preparation technique, a serving of brewed coffee usually contains between 60 to 150
mg of caffeine, while instant coffee typically has about 60 to 100 mg
of caffeine. Teas usually provide around 20 to 70 mg, and soft drinks
typically have approximately 35 to 55 mg of caffeine.[87,88]

Caffeine stimulates the nervous system, which results in the
release of epinephrine from the adrenal medulla as well as heart rate
and contractility elevations and peripheral vasodilation. Effects of
caffeine administration also include increased release of calcium from
the sarcoplasmic reticulum and elevations of cellular cyclic adenosine
monophosphate (AMP), which is responsible for the activation of the
hormone-sensitive lipase that results in the mobilization of fatty acids
from fat cells. Caffeine can also block adenosine receptors; adenosine
usually has a calming effect and blocking adenosine might partially
explain the stimulating effects of caffeine. It also acts as a mild
diuretic.

Due to the effects of caffeine on the nervous system, adipose
tissue, and skeletal muscle, it seems that caffeine has a positive influence on exercise performance. The common assumption is that since
caffeine increases fat mobilization from adipose cells, it will increase
fat utilization and therefore will spare glycogen stores during exercise,
which may extend exercise time. However, while higher levels of fatty
acids are often detected in plasma after caffeine ingestion, many
studies do not provide evidence for sparing glycogen. On the contrary,
glycogen depletion has been found to be similar with or without
caffeine consumption, which has led researchers to search for other
mechanisms responsible for the improvement in exercise performance.[89]

In an early study, 330 mg caffeine from coffee vs. a placebo were
ingested 1 hour before endurance performance.[90] Caffeine improved
performance significantly while enhancing fat use for energy. The
authors speculated that the increase in fat use decreased carbohydrate
use, thus allowing carbohydrate stores to supply energy later in exercise.

Another early study in which enhanced fat catabolism and reduced carbohydrate utilization apparently explained improvements in performance required participants to ingest 250 mg caffeine before exercise and an additional 250 mg every 15 minutes during exercise.[91]

There is inconsistency among some studies with regard to the dosage required to obtain improvements and the duration and intensity of exercise that will likely be affected. Some research suggests that the most effective dosage for improving exercise performance in intensities of about 80 to 85% VO_{2max} is approximately 9 mg of caffeine per kg body weight when this dosage is taken an hour before a competition.[87,92] In the research by Graham and Spriet, caffeine raised serum epinephrine concentrations and improved endurance running and cycling times.[92] The enhancement in epinephrine concentrations were theorized to be responsible for the improvement in performance. Past research suggests that an increase in circulating free fatty acids can decrease reliance upon carbohydrates for oxidation as a fuel for energy during exercise.[93]

Other researchers have detected no further benefit from caffeine consumption exceeding 5 mg per kg body weight.[94] In that study, cyclists consumed 5, 9, or 13 mg of caffeine per kg body weight for each of the three trials. Performance was equally improved for all trials. Some research has reported beneficial effects after ingesting as little as 3 mg of caffeine per kg body weight.[89] Most researchers demonstrating improvements have studied the effects of caffeine in runners or cyclists;[87] however, caffeine may improve swimming performance as well.[95]

Improvements in performance are likely limited to long-term endurance bouts of exercise. The majority of studies demonstrate that caffeine has no effect on exercise performance during incremental bouts lasting between 8 to 22 minutes or during bouts lasting less than 90 seconds.[87] Even though athletes such as weight lifters and throwers (discus, javelin, and hammer) have also been using caffeine as an ergogenic aid to enhance strength and power for many years, there are no studies available to describe any benefits for these athletes.

Caffeine consumption can have some side effects including insomnia, headaches, gastrointestinal disturbances, cardiac arrhythmias, and a stimulation of diuresis.[89] The diuretic effect of caffeine is of major concern especially when dehydration can be involved. Athletes participating in exercise conditions that might facilitate dehydration (such as long distances or in hot environments) are advised to increase their fluid intake and avoid any caffeinated drinks before the exercise.[89] However, some studies have revealed that consumption of caffeine did not have a different effect from water consumption on fluid losses or electrolyte imbalance even in hot conditions.[87]

Until January 2004, an Olympic athlete found to have urine caffeine of more than 12 mg per kg body weight (approximately 6 cups) was found to be guilty of doping and was banned from competing. However, since this rule was determined to be unfair toward coffee drinkers and since urinary caffeine is difficult to accurately detect after an endurance event (even after the consumption of large amounts of caffeine), the World Anti-Doping Agency requested to remove caffeine from the list of prohibited substances.[89]

Although many caffeine dosages have been studied, the majority of research studies consistently indicating performance enhancement have utilized doses of at least 300 mg approximately 1 hour prior to exercise. These doses may have some minor side effects including nervousness, restlessness, insomnia, and tremors, but it is not expected to cause long-lasting health impairment in most healthy, well-nourished individuals. A concern for endurance athletes is the potential dehydrating effect that can occur, since caffeine is also a mild diuretic, particularly to those not habituated to it. It has been demonstrated that a daily intake of caffeine less than 300 mg induces a mild diuresis that is similar to plain water. There is no evidence that this will result in an electrolyte imbalance that might endanger exercise performance or health when a typical U.S. diet is consumed. Sedentary people are even at lesser risk of dehydration from caffeine than athletes due to a smaller fluid loss via sweating.[87]

Calcitriol *See* **Vitamin D**

Calcium is a macromineral required in relatively large quantities from the diet. Foods rich in calcium include dairy foods such as milk, yogurt, and cheeses. Other foods that can provide reasonable amounts of calcium in the diet include sardines, legumes, green leafy vegetables (although spinach is a poor source due to a high oxalate content), and broccoli. Foods with added calcium such as fortified juices, bread and cereal products, and tofu set with calcium can be significant contributors to dietary intake.

Calcium has many important functions. The most obvious is for the production of healthy bones and teeth. Other functions include roles for muscular contraction, intracellular signaling, blood clotting, and activation of numerous enzymes integral for metabolism. Calcium is also important in maintaining normal blood pressure and decreasing the risk for colon cancer.

Dietary deficiency of calcium during youth can lead to rickets. In adults, calcium deficiency increases risk of developing osteoporosis.

Physical activity is also of primary importance for preventing osteoporosis. For more information about bone health in sports, see entries for osteoporosis, bone mineral density, and the female athlete triad.

Calorie is a term for a unit of measure for energy. One calorie is typically defined as the amount of heat required to raise 1 g of water by 1°C. The "joule" is often used internationally in place of the calorie, and one calorie is the equivalent of 4.184 joules. Nutritionists and dietitians usually refer to calories as Calories, which actually signifies kilocalories (kcal), since it would be cumbersome to refer to dietary energy or energy expenditure in calories.

Carbohydrates are macronutrients composed of carbon, hydrogen, and oxygen atoms and can be divided into many categories based upon their structure (i.e., monosaccharides, disaccharides, polysaccharides, and nondigestible polysaccharides) as well as their metabolic effects (such as digestibility, glycemic responses, and so forth). Many foods from each of the five major food groups, as well as sweets and foods specifically developed for athletes, can provide significant amounts of carbohydrates in the diet. Table C.1 provides some examples of carbohydrate-rich foods and their carbohydrate contents in 100 g servings. While many of the foods on the list appear to be rather low in carbohydrates, most of these foods have a high or very high water content, which can be misleading.

Dietary carbohydrates as well as endogenous carbohydrate production and metabolism, particularly during exercise, are critical issues for most athletes. Those athletes who should be particularly cognizant of their carbohydrate intake are endurance athletes, but most individuals utilizing high amounts of energy during training or competition are also likely to benefit from carbohydrate consumption. This book contains many carbohydrate-related entries in addition to this entry, which provides only a limited amount of information regarding carbohydrate and sports nutrition. For more details regarding specific issues, the reader is directed to entries for topics such as various individual carbohydrate molecules (for example, glucose, starch, trehalose, glycogen, etc.), carbohydrate loading, glycemic index, fiber, metabolic pathways of carbohydrate metabolism (for example, glycolysis, gluconeogenesis, Krebs cycle, etc.), interactions with dietary protein for muscle glycogen and protein synthesis, and several other topics found throughout this book.

Carbohdyrates are often classified structurally as either simple carbohydrates (typically monosaccharides and disaccharides) or complex carbohydrates (i.e., polysaccharides or starches). Monosaccharides are

C

carbohydrates composed of a single monomeric unit, while disaccharides include two monosaccharides linked by a glycosidic bond. The principal dietary monosaccharides are glucose, fructose, and galactose. Key disaccharides include sucrose (glucose + fructose), lactose (glucose + galactose), and maltose (glucose + glucose). Polysaccharides (also known as starches) include amylase and amylopectin. The structures of each of these carbohydrates are provided in their separate entries. Nondigestible polysaccharides (i.e., fiber) are also made of saccharide units, but are resistant to digestion by human enzymes. Fiber is described in separate entries.

Carbohydrates can also be categorized by how they affect metabolism. Currently, the most popular way to categorize digestible carbohydrates is based on the glycemic index, which is discussed in detail in a separate entry. Briefly, the glycemic index describes the impact that a food (usually rich in carbohydrate) has on the blood glucose response in the hours just after consumption. This can serve as a gauge for how quickly blood glucose is available for metabolism. It is currently being used to describe the ergogenic potential of some foods as well.

When a carbohydrate is ingested, it must be broken down by digestion to its simplest form prior to absorption, since the gut prefers to allow only the monosaccharides into the circulation. The blood circulating around the intestinal tract, where the monosaccharides are absorbed, is directed first to the liver. The liver is instrumental in converting nonglucose molecules into glucose derivatives that can either be metabolized further by the liver or released to the bloodstream. The vast majority of carbohydrate that is found within the blood is glucose, which provides a source of energy to most tissues of the body and is especially preferred by the red blood cells and tissues of the central nervous system. Furthermore, much of the energy produced within the skeletal and heart muscle is from glucose. When energy production is not required, glucose can be stored within the body, particularly in the muscle cells and liver, for future use.

The metabolic processes that are ultimately responsible for the production of energy from glucose include glycogenolysis, glycolysis, the pyruvate dehydrogenase complex, Krebs cycle, and the electron transport chain. Catabolism of glucose for energy eventually produces energy, primarily as adenosine triphosphate (ATP), carbon dioxide, and water. The energy produced by carbohydrate metabolism is critical for the muscle contraction of the body needed during the performance of exercise.

C

TABLE C.1
Typical Carbohydrate Content of 100 g Servings of Selected Foods and Sports Products Rich in Carbohydrate*

Food	Carbohydrate Content (g)
Bread, Cereal, Rice, and Pasta Group	
Bagels (plain)	50–55
Brown rice (cooked)	24
Cooked cereal (prepared with water)	10–20
Corn tortillas (unfried)	47
Crackers (saltine)	72
English muffins	46
Flour tortillas	56
Noodles (egg, cooked)	25
Pancakes	37
Pasta	25–30
Pretzels	79
Ready-to-eat cereal (dry)	80–90
Waffles	33
White bread or toast	50–55
White rice	29
Whole wheat bread or toast	47–51
Vegetable Group	
Corn	20
Peas	16
Potatoes (baked)	21
Yam (boiled)	28
Fruit Group	
Canned fruits	5–30
Dried fruits	60–80
Fruit juices	10–15
Raw fruits	15–25
Milk, Yogurt, and Cheese Group	
Cheese (fat free, processed)	13
Chocolate milk (low-fat)	10
Ice cream (fat free)	30
Milk (fat free)	5
Yogurt (fat free with fruit)	19
Meat, Poultry, Fish, Dry Beans, Eggs, and Nuts Group	
Chestnuts (roasted)	53
Dry beans (boiled)	23–27
Lentils	20

(continued)

C

TABLE C.1 (CONTINUED)
Typical Carbohydrate Content of 100 g Servings of Selected Foods and Sports Products Rich in Carbohydrate*

Food	Carbohydrate Content (g)
Sweets*	
Candy	80–98
Candy bar	60–70
Cookies (low-fat/fat free)	70-80
Honey	82
Jam/preserves	69
Maple syrup	67
Soft-drinks	10–11
Table sugar	100
Sports products*	
Sports bars	65–75
Sports drinks	5–7
Sports gels	70–80

* Information obtained from USDA National Nutrient Database for Standard Reference, Release 16-1.
** Usually low-nutrient density.

Dietary intake of carbohydrates should be considered relative to overall consumption during training as well as intake prior to, during, and after an event or rigorous training session. Adequate carbohydrate intake before and during an event is particularly effective for enhancing performance. Activities that are most likely to be affected by carbohydrate intake include: 1) rigorous endurance events lasting approximately an hour or longer; 2) events that include intermittent bursts of high-intensity activity; and 3) events performed in cold environments.[96]

Several studies have indicated that exogenous (dietary) carbohydrates provide an alternate fuel source that can spare the use of the body's glycogen reserves, thus prolonging the time to fatigue. This is particularly important given the relatively low amount of energy (~2000 kcal) that can be stored within the muscle and liver as glycogen.[97] A comprehensive review of the literature surrounding carbohydrate supplementation and performance is beyond the scope of this book; however, a review by Jacobs and Sherman summarizes much of the research regarding the efficacy of carbohydrates in optimizing endurance performance.

C

Research by Sherman and his colleagues has demonstrated in several studies that carbohydrate consumption prior to exercise can improve performance.[98,99] Furthermore, Coyle, Below, and their colleagues have demonstrated significant improvements in endurance in well-designed studies evaluating the roles of carbohydrate feedings during exercise in optimizing performance.[100,101] When carbohydrates were fed both prior to and during exercise, performance was improved to a degree greater than either feeding protocol alone.[102] As described in the protein entry, some research has also suggested that incorporating protein or essential amino acids into the foods consumed during exercise may be beneficial,[103] although this research has been criticized for lack of energy intake control among trials.

Adequate daily carbohydrate intake also appears to be important for maintaining the body's glycogen stores during periods of training,[104] although all research is not in agreement that performance is affected by regular consumption of a high carbohydrate diet. Some research has even suggested that a usual diet rich in fat may be more beneficial than a high carbohydrate diet.[105] If this is true, it may be possible that adaptation to a fat-rich diet during training and then a shift to a carbohydrate-rich diet for competition could prove to be optimal. More information about this topic is provided in the entry for fat loading.

Carbohydrate intake after exercise also appears to be important from the perspective of maximizing restoration of lost glycogen stores. Research suggests that carbohydrate-rich foods should be consumed soon after exercise to maximize the rate of glycogen synthesis.[106] Furthermore, while some research also suggests that incorporating protein/amino acids into the postexercise meal will stimulate additional glycogen synthesis,[107] not all studies are in agreement.[108] Interestingly, however, the combination of intake of carbohydrates and either proteins or essential amino acids after exercise may help to stimulate muscle synthesis after resistance exercise.[109]

Although carbohydrate needs vary by sport or event, timing of intake relative to competition or training, and individual athletes' preferences, basic guidelines for intake have been published.[96] The following guidelines apply most specifically to events or training sessions that are prolonged and rigorous in nature. A basic recommendation for carbohydrate consumption prior to an event is to consume 4 to 5 g/kg about 4 hours before the event begins. The athlete should experiment with different food sources, possibly including commercial carbohydrate supplements, to determine which foods will work best to achieve their goal intake level and optimal performance.

Closer to the event, when approximately 1 to 2 g/kg is consumed 1 hour prior to the event, it may improve performance, and feedings of 50 to 60 g/kg immediately prior to the event may prolong endurance. During an event it is generally recommended that athletes consume approximately 8 oz of a 5 to 10% carbohydrate solution every 15 minutes. This schedule is clearly not possible for all sports and events and should be adjusted for individual athletes in a manner that is appropriate for his or her particular competition.

The source of the carbohydrate selected to enhance performance is likely a secondary factor for most athletes. While most research suggests that the type of carbohydrate has relatively little impact, some research indicates that different sources may produce varying effects on the body's physiology and performance. For example, as described in the entry for the glycemic index, foods that promote a slower uptake of carbohydrate from the gut may be effective in enhancing performance relative to higher glycemic index foods when eaten in the period of about 15 to 60 minutes before exercise for some athletes.[110,111] Some researchers have also speculated, although adequate research is not available to support it, that foods promoting a faster entry of carbohydrates into the bloodstream may prove useful during and after an event. More research is needed to determine what type of carbohydrate is best for various occasions.

Carbohydrate loading (also known as glycogen loading), has been demonstrated to provide an advantage for performance for some athletes participating in prolonged endurance events. As the name implies, carbohydrate loading is a process in which the athlete consumes high levels of dietary carbohydrates in the days preceding an event. These carbohydrates maximize the storage of carbohydrate (glycogen) in the muscle and liver. A recommended technique for achieving the goal of loading the muscle and liver with glycogen includes tapering the volume of exercise during several days preceding the event. At this time, carbohydrate intake should comprise of approximately 70% of the energy in the diet. Restricting energy intake is not advised during carbohydrate loading, since the total grams of carbohydrate consumed would likely be insufficient to maximize glycogen storage. Additionally, early methods of carbohydrate loading that required a period of carbohydrate restriction and glycogen-depleting exercise in the period prior to loading are not recommended, since the final outcome of carbohydrate loading is similar between the two methods, yet the risk of adverse effects is greater when incorporating a depletion phase.

Carbohydrate loading clearly increases muscle glycogen content and can be effective for enhancing endurance in events of a prolonged

C

nature[112] or perhaps even in events that are shorter and performed at high intensities.[113] Athletes should experiment during training to determine if carbohydrate loading works for their particular sport.

Some athletes have reported some minor side effects that can be either unpleasant or may impair performance. These include gastrointestinal discomfort, weight gain, sluggishness, cramping, and related effects. Weight gain occurs due to increased retention of water that is stored along with the glycogen in the tissues. Additionally, although no research exists on carbohydrate loading in bodybuilders, some athletes have claimed that the extra water increases muscle volume, providing a larger appearance. Others have suggested that the water retention can cause the muscles to appear less defined and smoother in appearance. Overall, individual athletes should decide whether or not carbohydrate loading is beneficial or detrimental to their performance.

Sports dietitians, coaches, athletic trainers, and other practitioners should be aware of the foods and commercial products that can best provide the athlete with the carbohydrates needed to achieve this level of dietary intake. In general, nutrient-dense foods from the bottom three levels of the Food Guide Pyramid should be the focus of dietary intake during carbohydrate loading. Table C.1 provides a list of several sources of carbohydrate-rich foods that can be incorporated into the athlete's diet.

Carnitine The physiologically active form, L-carnitine (Figure C.1), is a water-soluble vitamin-like compound synthesized in the body and present in relatively high concentrations in skeletal muscle and in the heart. Carnitine is also supplied from the diet, primarily via animal protein sources (i.e., red meats, chicken, fish, eggs, and milk). The average nonvegetarian adult consumes 100 to 300 mg per day in their diet.[114] When dietary intake is low, such as in vegetarian diets, the body seems to compensate by increasing carnitine biosynthesis and decreasing renal clearance.[115,116] Once carnitine is formed in the body or ingested, the compound is released into the circulation and subsequently assimilated into the muscle, where it may impact both aerobic and anaerobic energy production during exercise.

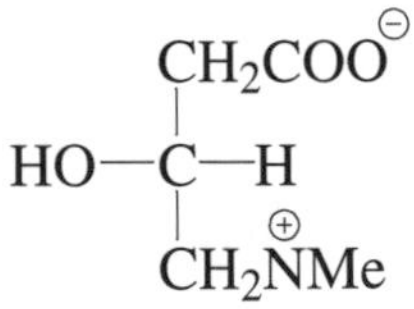

$$CH_2COO^{\ominus}$$
$$HO-C-H$$
$$CH_2NMe^{\oplus}$$

carnitine

FIGURE C.1

The primary function of carnitine involves the transfer of long-chain fatty acids across the mitochondrial membrane, where they are then oxidized. It has been hypothesized that increased availability of

C

carnitine to the muscle will increase fatty acid transport into the mitochondria, thus enhancing lipid oxidation during exercise.[114] As a result, reduced glycogen degradation may occur, potentially leading to prolonged endurance. Carnitine is also involved in the conversion of acetyl-CoA into acetyl-L-carnitine and CoA, which may favorably influence the citric acid cycle and decrease lactate accumulation during exercise.

Carnitine presumably enhances lipid oxidation, increases VO_{2max}, and decreases plasma lactate accumulation during exercise, which would lead to improved performance. Most carnitine studies, however, do not support its use for ergogenic purposes. Although several researchers have observed an increase in plasma carnitine concentrations with the administration of carnitine, few studies have reported changes in muscle carnitine values due to supplementation.[117] Interestingly, supplementation with choline may enhance carnitine availability for incorporation into tissue.[118] Other studies indicate no effect on muscle carnitine levels with carnitine supplementation.[119–121] While nearly all studies agree that carnitine supplementation does not directly improve performance, a few studies have revealed some positive effects on performance-related variables, suggesting possible metabolic shifts that would prolong endurance. Alternatively, researchers have suggested that endurance training may be related to increased endogenous synthesis of carnitine.[122]

Several studies have demonstrated no difference in various performance variables, including heart rate, lactate, running or swimming performance, and rating of perceived exertion (RPE) with carnitine supplementation.[122–131] A rather small trial, however, did find carnitine, especially when coingested with caffeine, to significantly enhance endurance performance.[132]

The dosing regimen that can maximize the potential for carnitine to enhance performance is unclear. A minor amount of studies have assessed the acute effect of carnitine ingestion on exercise performance. Most studies have provided 2 to 4 g of carnitine for 1 to 12 weeks. These regimens typically have no effect on endurance performance; thus, if carnitine has the potential to prolong endurance, some other dosing regimen is likely required. Recent studies also suggest that carnitine is ineffective in improving anaerobic athletic performance. Therefore, any reports of the efficacy of carnitine in improving sport performance remain largely based on theory.[114]

Carnitine supplements appear to be safe for consumption. Previous studies have reported few adverse effects of carnitine supplementation with dosages ranging from 500 mg/day to 6 g/day for periods of 1 to 28 days.[114] In summary, current available research indicates that carnitine supplementation appears to have little effect on the rate of fatty acid oxidation, muscle glycogen utilization, or sport performance.

Carotenoids are a group of plant chemicals (phytochemicals) that are yellow-orange pigments. They have antioxidant potential and many can be converted to vitamin A. As antioxidants, carotenoids may be important in reducing oxidative stress, which can be valuable for reducing muscle damage during exercise as well as protecting athletes from the development of chronic diseases that are promoted by oxidative stress. See the entries for beta-carotene and antioxidants for more information.

Catabolism refers to metabolic processes in which biomolecules are broken down. For example, catabolism of macronutrients produces water, carbon dioxide, and energy. The energy produced can be harnessed to drive chemical reactions within the body.

Catalyst A catalyst is a substance, such as an enzyme, that promotes in a chemical reaction but is not a reactant or a portion of the product.

Cation A cation is an ion with a positive charge. The term ion refers to a chemical that has either a positive or negative charge.

Cellulose (Figure C.2) is a nondigestible polysaccharide that is characterized by multiple glucose units linked by beta-1,4 glycosidic bonds. While cellulose is usually considered inert, colonic bacteria possess a limited ability to ferment it, producing short-chain fatty acids that can be absorbed by the colonic epithelium, thereby providing energy to the body. While some of the short-chain fatty acids absorbed into the intestinal cell can be transported to the circulation for uptake by the liver or peripheral tissues, they also provide a direct valuable energy source for the intestinal cells.

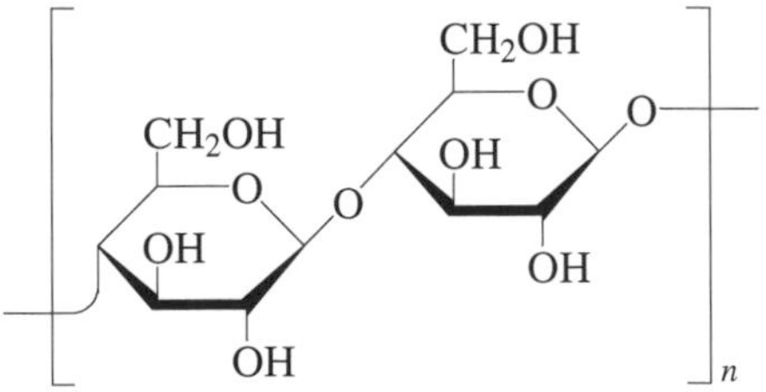

cellulose
FIGURE C.2

Central fatigue theory Scientists have theorized that since branched-chain amino acids (BCAA) are used extensively by muscle tissue for energy during exercise, the subsequent drop in plasma concentrations of BCAA combined with the displacement of tryptophan from albumin by an increase in concentration of free fatty acids can result in perceived exertion and thus premature fatigue. Tryptophan more readily enters the brain when the ratio of tryptophan to BCAA in the blood is elevated. Serotin production increases when tryptophan enters the brain, which may produce the sensation of fatigue and decrease an individual's ability to send a signal from the brain to the muscle for contraction.[80] This process has been referred to as the central fatigue theory.

Central fatigue is most likely to occur when levels of glycogen, a primary source of glucose and fuel for endurance exercise, become depleted. Glycogen depletion increases the body's reliance on BCAA and free fatty acids as fuel for working muscles, resulting in an increase in the ratio of tryptophan to BCAA in the blood, which allows for the increased uptake of tryptophan by the brain. Many researchers have attempted to improve performance by limiting central fatigue through BCAA supplementation, which is described in a separate entry. Research, however, better supports the consumption of carbohydrates prior to and during exercise as the most effective means of delaying central fatigue and improving performance. This can be the result of glycogen-sparing, producing less BCAA uptake as well as somewhat blunting the release of free fatty acids from the adipose tissue, so less tryptophan is displaced from albumin.[80]

Central nervous system (CNS) The central nervous system includes the brain and spinal cord in vertebrate animals.

Children *See* **Young athletes**

Chloride is the most abundant extracellular anion. Most of our dietary chloride is provided by salt (NaCl); however, chloride is also present in foods such as seafood, dairy foods, meats, and eggs. Many of chloride's functions are related to those of sodium, the extracellular cation whose charges are negatively opposed by chloride. Chloride is also a part of hydrochloric acid (HCl); thus, it is critical for digestion and for destroying pathogens that enter the stomach. Chloride also exchanges with the bicarbonate anion (HCO_3^-) in red blood cells in the process of delivering carbon dioxide (CO_2) to the lungs.

As a major electrolyte, when sweat losses are great, chloride losses will be high as well. While more attention has been given to the importance of adequate sodium and potassium during prolonged exercise, excess chloride loss can also produce an electrolyte imbalance. Electrolyte replacement fluids such as sports drinks typically provide sodium, potassium, and chloride. The importance of electrolyte

C

replacement during strenuous prolonged exercise is discussed in the entry on electrolytes.

Cholesterol As a member of a class of molecules referred to as sterols, cholesterol (Figure C.3) is a four-ringed steroidal structure with a single alcohol group. Dietary sources of cholesterol are limited to animal products; thus, nonanimal foods are cholesterol free unless they are prepared with an animal product. Foods rich in cholesterol include meats and organ meats, egg yolk, some dairy foods, and some seafood. Since the body's cholesterol needs can be met through biosynthesis, there is no dietary requirement for cholesterol.

Cholesterol is vitally important for life. Steroid hormones, vitamin D, and bile acids are synthesized from cholesterol, and it is an integral part of cellular membranes. Despite these critical functions, the general public perceives cholesterol as a threat, due to the relationship between elevated serum cholesterol and the risk for cardiovascular diseases.

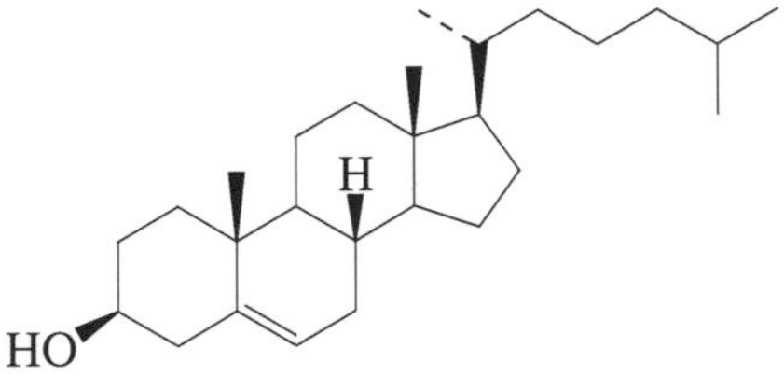

cholesterol

FIGURE C.3

Interestingly, exercisers typically have lower serum cholesterol concentrations compared to nonexercisers[133] and are at lower risk for heart disease.[134] Many studies have also demonstrated that exercise training will produce a cholesterol-lowering response in previously untrained individuals.[133] Typically, total serum cholesterol concentration as well as low-density lipoprotein cholesterol (cholesterol that is atherogenic) decreases with physical activity and the concentration of high-density lipoprotein cholesterol (which reduces heart disease risk) increases.[133]

Research has demonstrated that both resistance training and aerobic exercise can have favorable effects on serum cholesterol concentrations; however, aerobic exercise appears to be the more effective of the two.[133] In aerobically trained athletes, several studies have even suggested that exercise may blunt the adverse effects of a diet rich in saturated fat on serum cholesterol concentrations.[135,136] While this is

C

good news for the athlete, it should not send the message that athletes can eat any diet they wish with no risk of disease. There are many other risk factors for heart disease and research relating to the adverse effects of a diet rich in saturated fat on risk factors for other diseases (such as cancer, etc.) has not been conducted in athlete-specific populations.

Choline (Figure C.4) is an extremely important molecule that is now considered a vitamin by many scientists. In fact, the Food and Nutrition Board of the National Academy of Sciences has established Dietary Reference Intake values for choline, although endogenous synthesis can account for choline needs in many individuals.

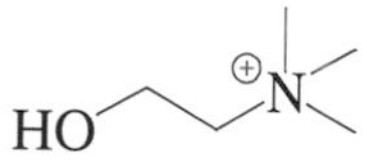

choline

FIGURE C.4

Phosphatidyl choline (a phospholipid also known as lecithin) is produced from choline and is a major part of cell membranes. It also participates in important metabolic processes, including the reverse cholesterol transport system, in which cholesterol is transferred to high-density lipoprotein cholesterol. Choline is also a component of acteylcholine, an important neurotransmitter found at the neuromuscular junction.

Choline and lecithin have been marketed for their ergogenic potential, primarily due to choline's association with acetylcholine and muscular contraction. While choline deficiency in those unable to produce adequate amounts of choline will almost certainly prevent optimal athletic performance, no studies have established a true ergogenic effect from choline or lecithin supplementation. Interestingly, as discussed in the entry on carnitine, when choline and carnitine are supplemented together, carnitine status increases, which may suggest that the combination is more likely to produce an ergogenic benefit or other physiological responses than either supplement alone.

Chromium is a micromineral found in a variety of foods including mushrooms, nuts, whole grains, asparagus, and beer. The primary function of chromium is as a component of the glucose tolerance factor along with niacin. This important complex has a critical, although not particularly well understood, role in the function of insulin; thus, chromium is vitally important for normal metabolism. Deficiency of chromium produces decreased insulin function, which produces glucose intolerance and altered lipid metabolism. The entry for insulin provides an overview of many of its important functions.

Due to chromium's essential role in insulin function, along with research suggesting that many Americans do not consume adequate amounts of chromium, some have speculated that chromium

C

supplementation (such as chromium picolinate) may increase lean body mass and strength as well as promote the loss of body fat.[137,138] Initial research reported an increase in body weight during 40-day and 12-week training programs, respectively.[137] In the Hasten study, no treatment effects were observed on strength, skin fold, and circumference measurements.[138] However, there was a statistically significant increase in body weight in female weight lifters, but no change in male weight lifters. It was not clear from the study if the weight gain was from increased fat or lean body mass. The results of the Hasten study have been questioned since the increase in body weight was reported only in females. The results are also questioned because the authors reported an increase in fat free mass, but not an increase in strength. Body weight was measured with the subjects wearing shorts, T-shirt, and tennis shoes, but there was no mention as to whether the researchers required the subjects to wear the same clothing and shoes for each of the 3-week measurements. The results of the Evans' study (see reference 137) are questioned because the subjects were poorly controlled during the training program, and there was no standardization regarding prior weight training experience.

A review of the majority of research available on healthy, active humans suggests that chromium is not effective as a fat-loss supplement.[139-145] These studies ranged from 8 to 14 weeks in duration and included a training program with chromium supplementation, which in each case failed to provide any additional benefits over training alone. Additionally, a study by Grant and his colleagues reported that chromium supplementation without training may result in an increase in body weight.[146] In this study, a group of nonexercising obese women gained almost 2 kg of body weight over a 9-week period. However, the researchers reported that a chromium nicotinate supplement in combination with a 9-week exercise training program with obese women resulted in an approximate 1 kg weight loss. This was the first statistically significant weight loss effect reported with chromium nicotinate.

The researchers also found that an exercising placebo group and an exercising group consuming a chromium picolinate supplement did not experience any change in body weight, fat free mass, or fat mass during the 9-week period. It is not known why the chromium picolinate group did not respond as well as the chromium nicotinate group. Although a statistical significance was found with chromium supplementation, these results are clearly in the minority of published research. There is little evidence from well-designed studies that show that chromium increases lean body mass or decreases body fat. In addition, research does not support the hypothesis that athletes require additional chromium in their diets because of increased losses from exercise. Overall, there is currently no evidence that chromium supplements are anabolic or have other benefits for healthy athletes.

Citric acid (or citrate), is an intermediate molecule in the citric acid cycle also known as Krebs cycle or the tricarboxylic acid cycle for the catabolism of macronutrients for energy. Citric acid is also found naturally in foods and is used as a chemical additive for tartness or to adjust food pH. Some research has evaluated the potential of citrate to improve performance as described in the entry for sodium citrate.

Citric acid cycle *See* **Krebs cycle**

Citrus arantium The purported effects of citrus arantium by purveyors of this herb are increased fat oxidation and greater body fat loss. The suggested active ingredient in these preparations is the compound synephrine. Neither citrus arantium nor synephrine have been well-studied regarding their potential influence on exercise performance.

Synephrine, a biogenic amine, appears to have stimulating metabolic effects somewhat similar to epinephrine; however, few modern studies have been conducted on this compound and even fewer regarding its oral administration. Data are not available to suggest that citrus arantium supplements can alter fuel metabolism in a way that could be related to enhanced athletic performance.

Ciwujia (*Radix Acanthopanax senticosus*) is an herb from China that has been marketed to enhance fat utilization and endurance performance in animals and humans. Well-designed research currently available does not provide any indication that ciwujia may alter metabolism in a way that can delay fatigue, however.[147,148] Until solid research supporting an ergogenic benefit is available, ciwujia cannot be recommended as an effective aid for performance.

CLA *See* **Conjugated linoleic acid**

CNS *See* **Central nervous system**

CoA *See* **Coenzyme A**

Cobalamin *See* **Vitamin B$_{12}$**

Cobalt is a mineral that forms part of the structure of vitamin B$_{12}$ (also known as cobalamins). No other nutritional functions of cobalt have been clearly identified.

Coenzyme The term coenzyme refers to a molecule that is required by an enzyme for function but does not participate directly in the reaction catalyzed by the enzyme. Some coenzyme molecules can participate with more than one enzyme.

C

Coenzyme A (CoA) (Figure C.5) is a molecule produced in part by pantothenic acid, which is part of its structure. The main functions of coenzyme A are to act as a donor and acceptor of acyl groups (such as fatty acids, etc.). For example, coenzyme A can accept or donate an acetyl group and in those capacities is critical for metabolic processes such as the Krebs cycle, beta-oxidation, fatty acid and cholesterol synthesis, and more.

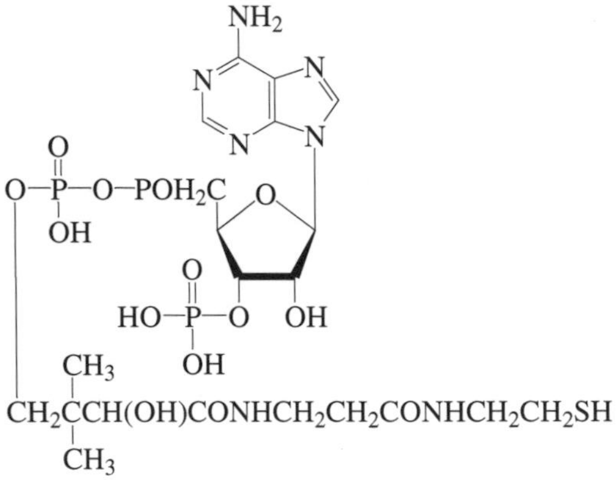

Coenzyme A

FIGURE C.5

Coenzyme Q (CoQ or CoQ$_{10}$) often referred to as coenzyme Q$_{10}$ or ubiquinone, is a natural compound produced endogenously that helps cells produce energy. CoQ$_{10}$ is essential for producing ATP by facilitating the transfer of energy stored in food through the electron transport system. As an antioxidant, CoQ$_{10}$ also helps protect and stabilize cell membranes.

While CoQ$_{10}$ is manufactured by the heart, liver, kidney, and pancreas, it also occurs naturally in some foods, most notably, organ meats, beef, eggs, and fish. However, various plant-based foods, such as whole grains, peanuts, and spinach, contain CoQ$_{10}$ in smaller amounts. As a fat-soluble compound, a small amount of oil or fat is needed for CoQ$_{10}$ to be effectively absorbed. CoQ$_{10}$ appears to be very safe as there have been no reports of significant toxicity in studies lasting up to 30 months.[149–151]

It has been hypothesized that supplemental CoQ$_{10}$ may enhance endurance and aerobic power due to its role in ATP formation and may be useful for athletes due to its antioxidant properties. Most research studies, however, have detected no improvement in performance indices. Studies report CoQ$_{10}$ supplementation (30 to 200 mg

C

daily) did lead to elevated plasma CoQ_{10} levels in a dose-dependent manner.[152] Other researchers have observed similar results on plasma CoQ_{10} levels.[153,154] Bonetti and colleagues reported no change in aerobic power following 8 weeks of CoQ_{10} supplementation, but results suggested an increased tolerance to higher workloads in the CoQ_{10} group.[155] No effect was observed in maximal oxygen uptake (VO_{2max}), submaximal physiological parameters, or lipid peroxidation in an 8-week trial where subjects consumed 100 mg daily of CoQ_{10}.[156] A shorter trial (22 days) also found no change in various performance parameters, including VO_{2max} determined during running, submaximal and peak VO_2, rating of perceived exertion, respiratory exchange ratio, blood lactate concentration, or heart rate determined during submaximal and maximal cycling between supplementation of 120 mg of CoQ_{10} per day vs. a placebo.[157] This research was further substantiated in a small double-blind, crossover placebo-controlled trial where athletes supplementing with 100 mg daily of CoQ_{10} demonstrated no effect on VO_{2max}, muscle energy metabolism or muscle fatigue.[153] Nevertheless, a Finnish study demonstrated that 90 mg of CoQ_{10} supplemented daily significantly improved aerobic threshold, anaerobic threshold, and maximal oxygen uptake.[158] Thus, according to the current literature, CoQ_{10} supplementation does not appear to enhance exercise performance or reduce oxidative stress induced by exercise.

Cofactor is a molecule that assists an enzyme in catalyzing a chemical reaction but does not participate directly in the reaction catalyzed by the enzyme. Some cofactors can participate with more than one enzyme.

Colon is another name for the large intestine.

Colostrum In recent years, bovine colostrum has been marketed as an anabolic supplement and ergogenic aid. Like human colostrum, bovine colostrum is the initial milk secreted by a mother just after birth. Colostrum is rich in many nutrients, and is especially known as a relatively rich source of biologically active compounds such as growth factors.

Available research has provided conflicting results regarding the efficacy of colostrum to enhance endurance as well as to increase lean body mass and strength.[159–163] While some research supports a role for colostrum in improving endurance[159] or sprint performance,[160] other studies have not provided similar evidence.[161–163] Likewise, while an increase in lean body mass[161] has been reported, increased strength has not,[161,162] and other research has failed to detect any changes in body composition.[160] Overall, more well-designed studies

C

are needed to determine the efficacy of colostrum and the potential mechanisms for its effects, if any.

Complementary proteins are foods that provide proteins that when eaten together supply all of the essential amino acids in proportions required to meet the demands for normal growth and development. Historically, protein complementation, the process of combining complementary proteins within a meal, was considered important for normal protein nutriture of vegetarians; however, most nutritionists now consider this process outdated and unnecessary as long as the individual is consuming a varied diet providing adequate total protein.

Complete protein A complete protein provides all of the essential amino acids at levels adequate to meet the demands for normal growth and development. Historically, all animal proteins, except gelatin, have been classified as complete proteins and all plant proteins, except soy protein, have been classified as incomplete proteins. The notion that plant proteins and gelatin are incomplete has been challenged, however, with opponents arguing that adequate consumption of many single plant foods could provide a profile of essential amino acids necessary to meet nutritional needs. Others argue that the classifications of complete vs. incomplete proteins are accurate, since in practical terms it would often be physically impossible to eat enough of some foods in order for humans to obtain enough of all of the essential amino acids. Furthermore, digestibility of the protein in foods should be considered when determining if a protein is likely to be complete. Most experts recommend that athletes consume a varied diet to ensure consumption of all essential nutrients, including essential amino acids, and foods providing high-quality proteins.

Complex carbohydrate is a digestible polysaccharide. The most prevalent examples of complex carbohdyrates in the human diet are amylose and amylopectin, both of which are considered starches. Many nutritionists have used the term complex carbohydrate to refer to foods rich in starches. These foods typically provide many nutrients other than the glucose that composes the starches and have long been considered to provide a nutritional advantage over simple sugars. Historically, this advantage has been used as a basis for suggesting that the diets of athletes be rich in complex carbohydrates. While many foods rich in complex carbohdyrates are also rich in nutrients, this is not always the case. Foods rich in complex carbohdyrates as well as fiber (such as whole grain breads, etc.) are examples of nutrient-rich foods that should form the basis of a healthy diet.

Concentric contraction is one in which the muscle shortens as it is contracted.

Conjugated linoleic acid (CLA) refers to a variety of isomers of linoleic acid containing conjugated diene units in which two double bonds are separated by only two carbons. The predominant isomer presents the double bonds of the fatty acid in the *cis*-9 and *trans*-11 positions.[164] CLA molecules are found in our foods, primarily in meat and dairy products. Average daily intake has been estimated to be approximately 150 mg for women and 200 mg for men.[165]

The potential influence of CLA on endurance exercise performance has not been formally studied. However, a 6-week study on CLA supplementation in bodybuilders was recently conducted.[166] This study was published only as an abstract in the proceedings at a national conference, and not as a peer-reviewed journal article. The researchers provided 7.2 grams of CLA vs. vegetable oil daily. The results suggested potential enhanced muscle growth via measurement of arm girth. This method of muscle growth measurement is highly questionable. Although this research does not suggest that endurance may be enhanced by CLAs, it does indicate that further high-quality research is needed to examine other potential ergogenic influences.

Research in mice indicates that CLA may stimulate norepinephrine-induced lipolysis.[167] This lipolysis results in the mobilization of free fatty acids from the adipose tissue to the bloodstream resulting in elevated plasma free fatty acids. An elevation in free fatty acids can result in enhanced fat oxidation and decreased utilization of carbohydrates for energy. Since these results have not been replicated in humans, this effect may be species specific.

Other studies have examined the effects of CLA on body composition. Some research has demonstrated no effect of CLA supplementation for a period of 28 days on lean body mass or strength.[168] Another study indicated that 3 g/day of CLA supplementation for 64 days did not alter body composition nor change energy expenditure or fat and carbohydrate utilization.[169] A well-designed study by Zambell et al. confirmed that 3.9 g of CLA each day for 64 days failed to alter fatty acid or glycerol metabolism of adult women.[170]

Much of the research involving CLA has centered on its potential roles for the treatment and prevention of diabetes mellitus. Insulin sensitivity may be improved through CLA supplementation, resulting in enhanced cellular uptake of glucose.[171]

Although long-term human studies of safety per se have not been conducted, no adverse incidents or toxicity effects due to CLA supplementation have been reported in the limited literature available. Overall, there is currently little research upon which to base a recommendation for CLA supplementation in athletes.

Copper is a micromineral that is essential in the diet. Dietary copper is obtained through many food sources but is most concentrated in organ meats such as the liver. More common sources include shellfish, whole grains, legumes, meats, fish, poultry, and nuts. Copper is required for a variety of functions, especially as a cofactor for many enzymes including several involved in the production of the protein collagen, which is essential for the development of connective tissue and bones. Copper also participates in the metabolism of tyrosine to various neurotransmitters and hormones. It is sometimes considered an anti-oxidant nutrient due to its activity with superoxide dismutase, an important antioxidant enzyme. Copper has not received serious atten-tion for potential ergogenic benefits, although a few, but not all, studies have demonstrated decreased copper status in athletes.[172]

CoQ *See* **Coenzyme Q**

CoQ$_{10}$ *See* **Coenzyme Q**

Cordyceps sinensis is an herb that has been used for centuries in China as a health stimulant. It is considered a bioactive compound with the purported ability to alter metabolism and has been used to treat mul-tiple conditions including lung, kidney, and cardiovascular problems as well as for body strengthening after illness or strenuous training. *Cordyceps* belong to the group known as "adaptogenic" herbs, which are considered to have antistress properties and enhance endurance and strength.[173] Although there are many claims regarding the effect of cordyceps on exercise performance, these reports are not supported by research. In a well-designed study that examined the effect of cordyceps on endurance exercise, no improvement in endurance was detected.[174]

Creatine (Figure C.6) is a naturally occurring nitrogenous compound that is consumed in the diet and produced in the body. An osmotically active substance, creatine is absorbed or synthesized in the liver, kid-neys, and pancreas from the amino acid precursors — glycine, methionine, and arginine. Once synthesized, creatine is

creatine

FIGURE C.6

transported to the muscle and heart via the bloodstream where it plays an integral role in energy metabolism. Dietary sources of creatine include meat, fish, and poultry. A mixed diet typically contains approximately 1.5 to 2.0 g creatine daily.[175] Oral ingestion of creatine naturally depresses biosynthesis of the compound. Nonetheless, indi-viduals following a vegetarian diet typically have lower intramuscular levels of creatine compared to nonvegetarians.[176,177]

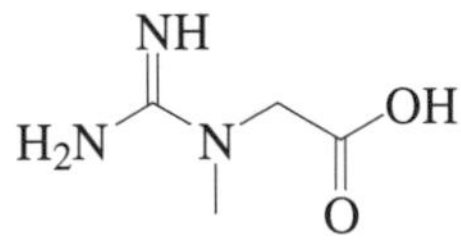

C

Ninety-five percent of the total creatine content is located in skeletal muscle while the remaining 5% can be found in the heart, brain, neural tissues, and testes. Thirty-three to forty percent of the total creatine pool exists in its free form while the remainder subsists in a phosphorylated form as phosphocreatine (PCr).[178] Once in the muscle cell, creatine and PCr remain there until creatine is metabolized. Creatinine, the end product of creatine metabolism, is generated via a nonreversible, nonenzymatic process.[179] This process occurs at a rate of 2% of the body's total creatine pool per day. Creatinine is then filtered in the kidneys and ultimately excreted in the urine.

During most exercises, ATP is provided through oxidative phosphorylation in the mitochondria. When energy demands exceed the capabilities of the oxidative delivery processes, which occurs during anaerobic activities, PCr is needed to form a much greater share of the ATP produced. The resynthesis of ATP from adenosine diphosphate (ADP) and PCr occurs more rapidly than glycogenolysis and glycolysis. This rephosphorylation of ADP supplies a considerable amount of energy during short-duration, high-intensity exercise.[175,179] Additionally, PCr has been proposed to function as a shuttle for the transport of high-energy phosphates between the mitochondria and the ATP utilization sites within the skeletal muscle cells.[180] Research has demonstrated that dietary and supplemental creatine can produce increased muscle PCr and total creatine content.[181–184]

The normal tissue content of creatine is maintained in the body at about 90 to 160 mmol/kg of dry matter.[175] The upper limit of creatine storage appears to be approximately 160 mmol/kg of dry matter. A 20-g daily dose of creatine for 5 days can produce a 15 to 40% increase in muscle creatine that can remain elevated for about 3 weeks.[175,185,186] Although somewhat common, currently low-dose supplementation (3 g for 30 days) seems to be less effective. The suggested loading dosage for creatine is 20 to 25 g per day for 5 or 6 days, followed by a maintenance dosage of 2 to 5 g daily. Creatine recommendations can also be adjusted by body weight to be about 0.3 g/kg/day during the loading phase, followed by 0.03 g/kg/day during the maintenance phase. Of note, research indicates that creatine supplementation may be of even greater benefit to vegetarians due to the lower levels of intramuscular creatine in vegetarians.[176]

Although the effects of creatine supplementation on sports performance have varied, more than 200 studies have observed statistically significant favorable effects.[187] No study reports a statistically significant ergolytic effect. Creatine supplementation accelerates the rate of ATP resynthesis following repeated bouts of high-intensity exercise. Creatine loading is said to improve exercise performance for rowing, running, cycling, swimming, and resistance type exercises, such as weight lifting. It has been demonstrated, however, that creatine serum, unlike creatine monohydrate powder, did not improve cycling sprint performance.[188]

Creatine supplementation does not seem to improve performance of endurance activities. In those types of events, normal PCr levels are considered to be sufficient to maintain adequate ATP levels.[175,189] Creatine exhibits greater effects in short-term, high-intensity intermittent exercises where ATP, PCr, and intramuscular glycogen stores are the primary energy supply. A recent review reported that the effects of creatine on muscle strength and weight lifting performance (maximal repetitions at a given percent of maximal strength) were greater when combined with resistance training compared to resistance training alone.[190]

Studies have indicated that creatine supplementation may increase total body weight or lean body mass possibly due to fluid retention or stimulating protein synthesis.[189] The increase in total body mass from short-term creatine supplementation is approximately 0.7 to 1.6 kg.[175] The change in body mass appears to be consistent in both males and females. Recent research has demonstrated that creatine supplementation, perhaps through increased water retention, may decrease the thermal burden of exercise performed in the heat.[191] These results were not confirmed by a recent similar study.[192] If creatine possesses this capability, it may be useful in preventing dehydration and heat stress, which can cause a decline in endurance performance.

Although more research is needed to understand the long-term effects of creatine supplementation, creatine appears to be rather safe. Gastrointestinal side effects, such as nausea, vomiting, and diarrhea have been reported only in an anedoctal manner.[193] Other studies, however, have failed to support these observations.[194]

Overall, current literature suggests that creatine supplementation increases total muscle creatine stores and PCr stores and improves maximal power/strength and improved performance in repeated bouts of exercise of an intense nature. It is possible that this could be useful to endurance athletes who participate in sports that include intermittent bursts of power that require quick recovery. This area is not well researched, however. When supplementation is combined with exercise training, additional gains have been observed in regard to fat free mass and sport performance during short-duration, high-intensity activities.

Creatine monohydrate *See* **Creatine**

Creatine phosphate *See* **Creatine**

Creatinine is produced within the muscle during the catabolism of creatine. Twenty-four hour urinary creatinine excretion is often used as an indicator of somatic protein status.

Cyanocobalamin *See* **Vitamin B$_{12}$**

Cysteine Along with methionine, the amino acid cysteine (Figure C.7) is one of the sulfur-containing amino acids required for protein synthesis. Cysteine is a nonessential amino acid because it can be synthesized from methionine. Besides production of proteins, cysteine is notably one of three amino acids that produces glutathione, which functions with glutathione peroxidase as an antioxidant.

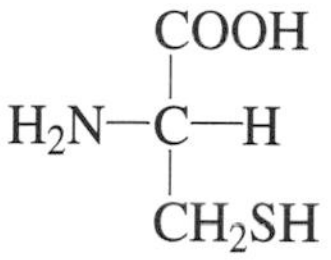

$$
\begin{array}{c}
COOH \\
| \\
H_2N-C-H \\
| \\
CH_2SH
\end{array}
$$

cysteine

FIGURE C.7

Cystine is an amino acid produced as a metabolite of cysteine. Although cystine is not incorporated into proteins within the body, it is formed within proteins by the joining of two cysteine thiol side-chains in the production of a disulfide bond. Disulfide bonds are important in determining a protein's conformation and providing stability to the structure.

D

Daily Reference Values (DRVs) are among the Daily Values (DVs) for nutrients established by the Food and Drug Administration. DRVs have been determined for total fat, saturated fat, carbohydrate, protein, fiber, cholesterol, sodium, and potassium. On a food label, the percentage of a nutrient met by a single serving of food is used to describe the nutrient content of that food.

Daily Values (DVs) are established by the Food and Drug Administration for food labeling and include the Daily Reference Values, or DRVs, and Reference Daily Intakes, or RDIs. Food labels describe the amount of a specific nutrient in a serving of a particular food as providing a certain percentage of the Daily Value, or DV, for that nutrient. For some nutrients (such as vitamins, minerals, protein, and so forth) the goal is to meet the DV for the average. For other nutrients (such as sodium, cholesterol, saturated fat, and so on) the goal is to keep the average day's intake below the established value.

Deficiency Nutrient deficiency occurs when the dietary intake of a particular nutrient does not meet the needs of the individual. For an athlete, a dietary deficiency is almost sure to result in a hindrance in athletic performance. Care, however, must be taken in evaluating scientific research that demonstrates improvement in performance when the nutritional status of an individual or a group is improved from a state of deficiency. This type of data does not demonstrate an ergogenic effect of a nutrient, but merely indicates that at least adequate status of that nutrient is needed for optimal performance. Many marketers of nutrients as ergogenic aid have seized upon such research to base their claims.

Dehydration occurs when fluid intake fails to meet the level of fluid excretion. For athletes, dehydration can be a major detriment to performance as described in the entry for hydration.

Dehydroepiandosterone (DHEA) is a metabolic steroid precursor to testosterone. As such, it has received a great deal of attention as a potential ergogenic aid that could elevate circulating levels of testosterone and produce increases in lean body mass and strength. These effects have not been well-documented in peer-reviewed research, however. Research has demonstrated that supplementation of DHEA can produce elevations in serum concentrations of DHEA in older men[195] and increased concentrations of DHEA, testosterone, and other androgens in women.[195,196] These studies, however, do not support a role for DHEA in improving body composition. In other research, neither hormonal changes or body composition changes were produced in young and middle-aged resistance-trained men.[197,198]

Dextrose *See* **Glucose**

DHA *See* **Docosahexaenoic acid**

DHEA *See* **Dehydroepiandosterone**

Diabetes mellitus (DM) is a disease characterized by abnormal regulation of blood glucose. It can be classified as Type I DM (also known as juvenile or insulin-dependent diabetes) or Type II DM (also known as age-onset, obesity-related, or noninsulin dependent diabetes). Individuals with Type I DM produce little if any insulin and thus require exogenous insulin for regulation of normal blood glucose levels, while most people with Type II DM produce insulin but are resistant to its function.

Exercise is important for regulating blood glucose in individuals suffering from DM. Athletes must take care in timing exercise with their food intake and medication use to acheive good blood glucose balance. Although more thought is required for exercise timing during training and competition, DM does not necessarily prevent an athlete from achieving an elite level of training.

Dietary fiber   Fiber has been classified into two general categories: dietary fiber and functional fiber. Dietary fibers are nondigestible polysaccharides, as well as lignin, that are intrinsically present as intact fibers in plants. Functional fibers are also nondigestible by human enzymes, but can be found in the diet through means other than natural whole foods. See the fiber entry for a detailed description of fibers as well as their relevance to athletes.

Dietary Guidelines for Americans were developed by the United States' Departments of Agriculture (USDA) and Health and Human Services and were last revised in the year 2000 and are currently being updated. The entry on dietary recommendations for athletes includes an overview of the 2000 version.

Dietary Reference Intakes (DRIs) are established by the Food and Nutrition Board of the National Academy of Sciences. There are four components to the DRIs, which include Recommended Dietary Allowances (RDAs), Estimated Average Requirements (EARs), Adquate Intake values (AIs), and Tolerable Upper Intake Levels (ULs). Each of these values are described in detail within their corresponding entry.

Dietary recommendations for athletes While there are no substitutes for genetic endowment and rigorous training in the achievement of optimal athletic performance, sound nutrition is critical for maximizing athletic potential. The importance of adequate dietary intake for athletes has been recognized for centuries, yet the modern field of sports nutrition is still very young and much is yet to be learned about using foods and dietary supplements for achieving optimal performance. Although controversies persist with regard to how diet may provide a winning edge, few researchers or dietitians would argue against the concept that an inadequate diet, deficient in energy or essential nutrients, will impair performance.

D

The key to proper nutrition is consuming a natural, wholesome diet providing a variety of foods from each of the food groups. Consuming a balanced diet is important not only for optimizing performance, but also for the prevention of many chronic diseases, such as heart disease, stroke, cancer, and diabetes, which are related to poor eating practices. Many nutritional guidelines such as the Food Guide Pyramid and the Dietary Guidelines for Americans are available to the athlete, sports dietitian, athletic trainer, and coach to help with making wise food selections and designing diets. The 2000 edition of the *Dietary Guidelines for Americans*, published jointly by the United States Department of Agriculture and the United States Department of Health and Human Services, provides several sensible practices that can serve as foundations for healthy eating. These guidelines include the following:

1. Aim for Fitness
   - Aim for a healthy weight.
   - Be physically active each day.
2. Build a Healthy Base
   - Let the Food Guide Pyramid guide your food choices.
   - Choose a variety of grains daily, especially whole grains.
   - Choose a variety of fruits and vegetables daily.
   - Keep foods safe to eat.
3. Choose Sensibly
   - Choose a diet that is low in saturated fat and cholesterol and moderate in total fat.
   - Choose beverages and foods to moderate your intake of sugars.
   - Choose and prepare foods with less salt.
   - If you drink alcoholic beverages, do so in moderation.

The Food Guide Pyramid provides a more specific set of recommendations for consuming an adequate diet without excess intake of energy, fat, saturated fat, cholesterol, added sugars, sodium, and alcohol. The Pyramid was developed as a practical representation of food selection for the *Dietary Guidelines for Americans*. Although more specific than the basic dietary guidelines described above, a major strength of the Pyramid is that it allows the user a high degree of freedom to make selections that fit his or her personal tastes, beliefs, economic status, and other factors that affect dietary intake. The entry for the Food Guide Pyramid provides details regarding current specific recommendations for food intake for each group.

Dietary Supplement Health and Education Act (DSHEA) The DSHEA was signed into law in 1994. It allows supplement manufacturers to provide an array of dietary supplements to the public. It also prevents manufacturers from making unsubstantiated claims on supplement containers and labels. While DSHEA provides some protection to consumers, it has often been criticized for failing to establish more stringent rules for supplement manufacturers.

Dietary supplements are compounds that can be consumed in addition to an individual's general food intake. Supplements can include a wide variety of compounds and mixtures including vital nutrients such as vitamins, minerals, proteins, amino acids, lipids, essential fatty acids, or carbohydrates. Other dietary supplements include herbs and botanicals, or chemicals extracted from these sources, as well as molecules produced in metabolism such as hormone and nutrient metabolites. Dietary supplements are regulated by the Dietary Supplement Health and Education Act (DSHEA), which is described in the previous entry.

Athletes are constantly searching for a special food or dietary supplement that will offer an advantage, which will allow them to perform better than their fellow competitors. Substances that provide such advantages are referred to as ergogenic aids, in other words, they enhance performance. It is no surprise that manufacturers often market their dietary supplements with the athlete in mind; however, the majority of the claims made for substances marketed as ergogenic aids lack credible scientific evidence.

Each year sports teams and athletes spend millions of dollars on products that are marketed to enhance performance, which are not substantiated by research. Sports dietitians, coaches, and athletic trainers are often responsible for providing athletes with current and accurate information regarding the use of these products that more often than not fail to fulfill their claims. The majority of the time, research on the efficacy of most products is either unavailable, deficient in proper study design, or fails to provide any evidence of benefit.

D

However, research on some products does suggest that a few purported ergogenic aids may truly improve athletic performance.

While some dietary supplements have been demonstrated to improve athletic performance or produce metabolic responses that may impact performance, the majority of supplements marketed to athletes are unproven and are often marketed based on false or misleading claims. Without a doubt certain dietary practices can contribute to the success of an athlete. Even for supplements for which little or no research suggests a beneficial effect, there is always the possibility of either a real physiological or pharmacological effect that may be specific to the individual or sport in which the athlete is participating. There may be some positive psychological benefits as well. Alternatively, using a particular supplement may include adverse side effects, excessive expense, a false sense of security, or illegality. The challenge for practitioners who work with athletes is to provide the necessary information so that the athletes can put the practitioner's knowledge into practice and make informed decisions on the use of supplements. Practitioners and trainers should always consider the following three issues when assisting athletes with the use of dietary supplements: 1) legal concerns; 2) health risks; and 3) maintaining rapport with the athlete. These issues along with details on how to evaluate marketing claims of ergogenic prospects were well-reviewed by Butterfield.[199]

From a legal perspective, practitioners should recommend that athletes abstain from all substances considered illegal by state and federal laws or that are banned for use during competition. Although some of these substances can improve performance, legal and health complications far outweigh their benefits. Practitioners should remain current on which substances are banned and which commercial products include those substances. Some products may include a banned substance, yet be marketed as containing another; therefore, supplements should only be purchased from reputable manufacturers.

For substances that are not banned, health risks may still be a concern. Many products marketed as ergogenic aids possess health risks that are often not regulated by the Food and Drug Administration. Athletes and many practitioners often make the mistake of assuming that since a product is available for purchase it must be safe and effective. In reality, numerous products are thought to potentially cause a variety of health problems and many other products lack research on short-term and long-term health implications. The common phrase "buyer beware" is extremely appropriate when it comes to dietary supplements. Each athlete has the right to weigh

D

the potential benefits vs. the potential side effects when making his or her decision about using a supplement; however, the practitioner can often provide valuable information that will allow the athlete to make the best choice.

In addition to potentially producing direct impacts on health status, some products may have hazardous effects through replacement of natural, wholesome foods. The product selected may fail to provide the same nutrients that could have been obtained through the food that the athlete has given up in favor of the supplement. Excess use of such products may produce a nutritional inadequacy that could impair performance or adversely affect one's health. Although the product itself may not be directly causing harm, it may still be producing damaging effects.

As described by Butterfield, maintaining rapport with an athlete who is using a questionable dietary supplement that appears to be safe for consumption can be critical.[199] A good relationship with the athlete may allow the practitioner to provide valuable assistance that may otherwise be dismissed in the absence of such rapport. Rapport can be lost when the practitioner tells an athlete that he or she will obtain no benefit from a product that the athlete believes will work. Practitioners should keep in mind that some athletes are prone to the "placebo effect." These athletes may gain a benefit from a supplement simply by believing it will work. Furthermore, many athletes are sponsored by manufacturers of questionable supplements. Recommending that the athlete not use a supplement provided by his or her sponsor may strain the relationship between the practitioner and athlete. Additionally, on many occasions coaches or teammates suggest the use of specific supplements. Under such circumstances, allowing the use of ergogenic prospects that are likely safe is warranted to prevent problems for the athlete, team, or practitioner. As stated by Butterfield, "this year's ergogenic aid is next year's garbage."[199] So if there are valid reasons to allow an athlete to use a questionable supplement that is considered safe, such use will often be short-lived and without incident.

Overall, proper dietary intake can prevent performance decrements that occur with nutritional deficiencies or excesses. Dietitians or other practitioners should attempt to instill in their athletes the idea that following good dietary practices is an important component of an optimal training regimen. Athletes should adhere to basic dietary guidelines stressing a diet high in carbohydrates and fluids to ensure adequate intake of energy, nutrients, and water. Coaches, athletic trainers, and others working with athletes may wish to encourage athletes to consult a registered dietitian for professional help with regard to proper dietary selection. Practitioners should also bear in mind that although evidence suggests that a few dietary practices may enhance performance, most supplements are marketed without scientific research demonstrating product efficacy. These supplements should be used only after considering their safety and legality.

Dietitian *See* **Registered dietitian**

Diffusion is the movement of a substance (i.e., a solute in a solution) from an area of high concentration to an area of low concentration. When discussing nutrient absorption, diffusion is also called passive absorption.

Digestion The process of breaking down food in preparation for absorption is called digestion. While a portion of digestion includes chewing food, lubricating food with saliva, and grinding food within the stomach, complete digestion requires enzymatic or chemical digestion of nutrients in foods, such as macronutrients. This type of digestion occurs primarily in the small intestine. Overall, chemical digestion in the stomach is primarily limited to the actions of HCl, which denatures protein, and pepsin, which is responsible for breaking protein down into smaller polypeptide units. Within the small intestine, chemical digestion is accomplished by many digestive enzymes produced in the pancreas or by the small intestine itself.

Dimethylglycine *See* **Pangamic acid**

Dipeptide A dipeptide is two amino acids linked together by a peptide bond.

Disaccharide A disaccharide is a carbohydrate containing two monosaccharides linked by a chemical bond. Sucrose, lactose, and maltose are common dietary disaccharides.

Disordered eating *See* **Eating disorders**

Dispensable amino acid *See* **Nonessential amino acid**

Diuretic A diuretic is any substance that increases the production of urine and the loss of body water. Common chemicals in food that can produce a diuretic effect include caffeine and alcohol.

Docosahexaenoic acid (DHA) is a long-chain (22 carbons) omega-3 polyunsaturated fatty acid found primarily in fish oil. DHA is highly unsaturated with six double bonds. The potential role of DHA in athletic performance is described in the entry on omega-3 fatty acids.

DRIs *See* **Dietary Reference Intakes**

DRVs *See* **Daily Reference Values**

E

EAR *See* **Estimated Average Requirement**

Eating disorders are among the most concerning psychological disorders that affect athletes, particularly young women. An eating disorder may be defined as a persistent disturbance of eating behavior intended to control weight that significantly impairs physical and psychological functioning.[200] Eating disorders include anorexia nervosa, bulimia nervosa, and other disordered eating behaviors that include weight control behaviors as well as subclinical eating disorders.[201] Subclinical eating disorders or disordered eating behaviors include symptoms of eating disorders and serious body weight concerns, but fail to reach the strict diagnostic criteria for anorexia nervosa or bulimia nervosa according to the *Diagnostic and Statistical Manual of Mental Disorders (DSM-IV)* criteria.[202] A position stand by the American College of Sports Medicine defined disordered eating behaviors as "A wide spectrum of harmful and often ineffective eating behaviors used in attempts to lose weight or achieve a lean appearance. The spectrum of behaviors ranges in severity from restricting food intake to binge and purging, to the *DSM-IV* defined disorders of anorexia nervosa and bulimia nervosa."[203] The *DSM-IV* reports that at least 90% of individuals suffering from eating disorders are women; while males represent less than 10% of all cases.

The *DSM-IV* also reports that the onset of disordered eating behaviors usually occurs between adolescence and early adulthood and that the prevalence of anorexia nervosa and bulimia nervosa among young women is 0.1 to 1.0% and 1 to 3%, respectively. Furthermore, 1 in 100 females between the ages of 12 to 18 is anorectic and 8 to 19% of college women suffer from bulimia nervosa.[202] According to the *DSM-IV*, anorexia nervosa is characterized by a distorted body image, an extreme fear of gaining fat, and the refusal to maintain body weight over a minimal level according to age and height.

Anorectics restrict food and often exercise obsessively and might use other methods to lose weight such as diuretics, laxatives, and purging. Bulimia nervosa is characterized by repeating episodes of consuming a large amount of food (binge eating) while feeling lack of control over eating during those episodes. It also includes purging behaviors (self-induced vomiting), as well as the use of diuretics and laxatives. Those suffering from bulimia often engage in food restriction, compulsive exercise, and extreme concern about shape and body weight.[202] There are many potential medical complications that can result from disordered eating. Complications from anorexia nervosa include hypothermia, hypotension, edema, infertility, cardiac failure, electrolyte imbalance, and death. Some complications that can occur from bulimia nervosa include dental caries, laxative dependence, electrolyte disturbances, gastric rupture, cardiac arrhythmias, and chronic pancreatitis. Other complications include amenorrhea (menstrual dysfunctions) and loss of bone mass, which can lead to osteoporosis.[204] When athletes experience menstrual dysfunction and bone loss induced by disordered eating, the condition is referred to as the female athlete triad, which is described in more detail in a separate entry.

In recent years, athletic participation has been associated with a higher prevalence of eating disorders, including anorexia nervosa, bulimia nervosa, and other subclinical eating disorders and disordered eating behaviors. Athletes are usually considered to be healthy because of their active lifestyle. However, recent studies found that as a consequence of their level of commitment and competitive nature, they are more prone to engage in disordered eating behaviors in an effort to improve their performance. Some researchers suggest that because of the unique pressure associated with sports, such as performance and coaches' expectations, and because the sports environment represents one of the subcultures in which there are specific demands for a certain weight and physical appearance, athletes may engage in unhealthy eating behaviors that might lead to an eating disorder.[205] Some studies have shown that athletes are 2 to 3 times more likely than nonathletes to manifest characteristics of eating disorders.[204] Overall, the risk for developing disordered eating behaviors among female athletes ranges from 35 to 89% including high school, college, and elite competitors.[205–208]

Eating on the road During times of competition, athletes often experience the need to eat out while traveling. In many cases, such as in college and high school athletics, food choices can be limited by finances, time-constraints, and the coach's personal preferences. In other cases, the athlete has a wide array of choices from which to select his or her meals while on the road. An athlete must not only be concerned with satisfying his or her hunger, but also nutritional status, in order to ensure optimal sports performance. Eating on the road can create problems for the athlete, such as temptations for foods that do not contribute to optimal performance and a tendency to overeat. It is

E

TABLE E.1
Portable Snacks for Athletes

Sports bars	Granola bars	Whole-grain crackers	Carrot and celery sticks
Dried fruits	Trail Mix	Pretzels	Whole-grain bagels, bread, tortillas, and rolls
Graham crackers	Peanut butter and jelly	Canned tuna, sardines, salmon	Portable fruit, such as bananas, apples, oranges
Cereal	Popcorn	Single containers of applesauce, peaches, apricots, pears	Fig bars
Single-serve microwavable soups	Low-fat chips	Single-serve microwavable packets of oatmeal	Canned liquid meals

TABLE E.2
Healthy Snacks that Athletes Can Keep in Hotel Refrigerators for Eating on the Road

Low-fat or skim milk	Cottage cheese	Yogurt	Juice
Cereal, dry and hot (microwavable)	Cheese	Fresh fruits	Low-fat luncheon meats
Prewashed bagged salads	Salad dressing	Fresh vegetables	Low-fat pudding

possible to eat on the road and choose high-performance foods; however, it takes planning and practice.

The most common current sports nutrition recommendation of consumption of a low-fat, high-carbohydrate, high-nutrient density diet allows an athlete to maintain optimal energy levels and repair muscles. However, many foods from restaurants and convenience stores tend to be high in unhealthy fats and low in nutrients.

It is a good idea to prepare for the trip by bringing nutrient-dense foods that travel well. This will provide familiarity with favorite foods and prevent the temptation to visit convenience stores. When making stops at convenience stores, however, the athlete can use the microwave ovens and toasters that are often available for use by customers to prepare some of the items in Table E.1, which can be portable, nutritious snacks. Upon arriving at the place of competition, if a refrigerator and microwave are available, it is a good idea to stock up on nutritious foods such as those listed in Table E.2. Many combinations of these

E

TABLE E.3
Healthy Meals that Athletes Can Prepare from Portable Snacks and Readily Available Foods

Breakfast	Lunch	Dinner
Whole-wheat bagel	Bean and cheese tacos	Sandwich with luncheon meat
Peanut butter and jelly	Carrot sticks	Soup
Piece of fruit	Granola bar	Yogurt
Milk	Fresh fruit	Dried fruit
	Milk	Milk

simple and nutritious foods can create a quick breakfast, lunch, or dinner in the hotel room. Examples are included in Table E.3.

Restaurants often have lower fat items to choose from. Many restaurants, especially fast food and other chains, offer nutrition information brochures for all of their items. Athletes and coaches can use these to make informed dining decisions. If there are no foods on the menu that meet healthy guidelines, do not hesitate to ask the server to make simple changes to menu items to reduce the fat and increase the nutritional content. It is imperative to know what to look for and to keep general guidelines for dining out. The following are a few basic guidelines to consider:

- Select foods that are broiled, grilled, baked, steamed, or boiled rather than fried.
- Ask for extra vegetables on sandwiches and pizzas or have a side dish of vegetables instead of fries or chips.
- Choose barbecue sauce, ketchup, or mustard instead of mayonnaise for added flavor.
- Order low-fat milk or 100% juice instead of soda.
- Request salad dressing on the side to control the amount used.
- Ask for a side salad instead of fries in "value" meals.
- Ask how the meal item is prepared (how much butter or oil is used in the preparation of the meal). For example, when ordering a grilled chicken sandwich, find out if they put butter on the bun prior to toasting. If so, ask for it to be toasted without the butter.
- Ask for special sauces and toppings on the side, which provides the athlete with control over how much to add.
- Ask for less cheese on items such as pizza and Mexican food; add more vegetables.
- Sit-down restaurants often serve very large portions; split an entrée with someone else, and order a side salad.

TABLE E.4
Words on Restaurant Menus that Signal Foods Prepared with Fat

Fried or pan-fried	Scampi sauce
Crispy	Breaded or lightly breaded
Buttery or butter sauce	Sautéed
Creamed or creamy	Alfredo sauce
Sauce	À la king
Gravy	Scalloped
Au gratin	Fritters
Cheese sauce or stuffed with cheese	Hollandaise
Rich	Tempura
Béarnaise	Croquettes
Newberg	

E

- Avoid the temptation to order the "super" or "value" size meals. This will save hundreds of nonnutrient dense calories and many grams of fat. Complement the meal with water or milk and a side of salad or fruit.
- When reviewing a menu for choices, be aware of words that signal high fat preparations, such as those in Table E.4; and avoid choosing too many foods in the high and moderate fat food choice lists in Table E.5.
- Use Table E.6 to help make healthy selections at various types of restaurants.

Eccentric contraction is one in which the muscle lengthens as it is contracted.

Eicosanoids are a group of compounds that have hormone-like effects and are synthesized by cyclooxygenase and lipoxygenase enzyme systems from long-chain fatty acids. Eicosanoids are classified as thromboxanes, leukotrienes, or prostaglandins. The functions and potencies of eicosanoids vary among classifications and within each class depending upon which fatty acid is used for its synthesis. These functions include blood vessel or bronchiole dilation or constriction, platelet aggregation or antiaggregation, pro- or antiinflammatory responses, chemotaxis, and other roles.

Eicosanoids produced from omega-3 fatty acids have been theorized to produce ergogenic benefits in endurance athletes primarily by their ability to produce vasodilation and reduce platelet aggregation, thereby allowing increased blood flow and oxygen delivery to the tissues. However, there are no studies that have directly administered eicosanoids to determine if they provide a true ergogenic benefit.

As summarized by Williams, some researchers have fed supplements rich in omega-3 fatty acids and assessed potential benefits with little or no indication of an ergogenic effect.[209] For more information, see the entry for omega-3 fatty acids.

E

TABLE E.5

Foods that Are Commonly Found While Eating on the Road as Categorized by Fat Content

Lower Fat Choices	Moderate Fat Choices	High Fat Choices
Low-fat or skim milk	2% milk	Whole milk
Frozen yogurt	Soft-serve ice cream	Regular ice cream
Low-fat milk shakes	Milk shakes	Biscuit, croissant
Bagels, English muffins	Small order French fries	Hash browns
Pancakes, waffles	Cornbread	Large/Super order French fries
Cereals	Chicken or tuna salad	Curly, cheese, or other fries
Bread sticks, plain	Cole slaw	Pastry, pie, or brownie
Baked potatoes, plain	Macaroni or potato salad	Olives
Salad greens	Cheeseburger	Croutons
Carrot, celery sticks	Steak sandwich	Bacon bits
Pasta, plain	Bean and cheese burrito	More than 2 tbsp. of full-fat
Fresh fruit		salad dressing
Soups, not cream-based		Caesar salad with dressing
Low-fat dressings		Cobb salad with cheese and
Chicken filet		meat
Chicken fajitas		Cream-based soups
Grilled chicken sandwich		Fried chicken
Chili with beans		Fried fish
Hamburger, plain		Fried fish or chicken nuggets
Vegetable pizza		"Super," "Deluxe," or
Chicken/turkey/ham/roast		"Supreme" sandwich/burger
beef sandwich or sub		Sausage, pepperoni, or extra
Bean burrito		cheese pizza
Ketchup		Bacon burger
Mustard		Beef and cheese burrito
Barbecue sauce		Breakfast biscuits (egg with
		sausage, cheese, etc.)
		Sausage, bacon
		Mayonnaise
		Mayo-type sauce
		Alfredo sauce
		Hollandaise sauce
		Added butter or margarine

TABLE E.6
Meal Ideas at Various Styles of Restaurants*

Burger Joint	Sub Sandwich Shop	Italian Restaurant	Family-Style Restaurant	Mexican Food Restaurant
Single patty hamburger	6-inch chicken, roast beef, or turkey sub with mustard and vegetables	2 slices cheese and vegetable pizza	Rotisserie chicken breast with skin removed or lean grilled steak	Bean burrito with grilled vegetables
Side salad with low-fat dressing	Small bag of pretzels	Side salad with low-fat dressing 100% juice, water, or low-fat milk	Steamed vegetables and new potatoes	Salsa Water
Grilled chicken sandwich	6-inch tuna sub made with low-fat mayonnaise	Pasta with tomato sauce and vegetables	Bowl of chili or broth-based soup	Grilled chicken fajitas with vegetables
Small order fries	Baked chips	Garlic bread Side salad	Baked potato with small amount of sour cream Salad	Corn or flour tortillas

* Beverages could be water, 100% juice, or low-fat milk.

Eicosapentaenoic acid (EPA) is a long-chain (20 carbons) omega-3 polyunsaturated fatty acid found primarily in fish oil. EPA is highly unsaturated with five double bonds. The potential role of EPA in athletic performance is described in the entry on omega-3 fatty acids.

Electrolytes are electrically charged ions that include sodium, potassium, chlorine, calcium, and magnesium. Blood plasma and extracellular fluids mainly contain the minerals sodium and chlorine, while potassium is the main mineral in the intracellular fluid. Sodium and potassium have an important role across cell membranes. These electrolytes maintain an electrical gradient, which stimulates the transmission of nerve impulses, stimulates muscle contraction, and maintains gland activities.[210]

Water and electrolyte balance are critical for the function of all organs and for maintaining health in general. Physical exercise and heat conditions cause imbalances in both fluid and electrolyte concentrations. During exercise, inadequate fluid intake can lead a person to become dehydrated (hypohydration). Hypohydration increases physiologic strain and decreases exercise performance. Sodium chloride is the primary electrolyte in sweat, while potassium, calcium, and magnesium are present in smaller amounts. The sodium concentration in sweat averages 35 mmol/L (range: 10 to 70 mmol/L) and varies by diet, sweating rate, hydration, and degree of heat acclimation.[211]

Sweat glands reabsorb sodium by active transport, but there is no increased ability to reabsorb sweat sodium at the high rate of sweating that can occur during exercise; therefore, at high sweating rates the concentration of sweat sodium increases. The potassium concentration in sweat averages to approximately 5 mmol/L; the concentration of calcium is approximately 1 mmol/L; and that of magnesium is 0.8 mmol/L. Sex, maturation, and aging do not appear to significantly affect sweat electrolyte concentrations. [211]

Plain water is typically not considered the best fluid to ingest in order to replenish exercise-induced water loss. For effective rehydration, electrolytes should be replenished as well as water. When water alone is ingested, sodium concentrations may become diluted, which might progress to a state of hyponatremia (which can also occur with excessive hydration); however, when adding dietary sodium to water, plasma sodium concentrations are more likely to remain stable.[212] Sodium helps in maintaining plasma osmolality, which plays an important role in higher thirst perception.[212,213] As a result, the levels of the hormones vasopressin and aldosterone are maintained, which results in reduced diuresis.

Several studies have determined that urine production during exercise decreases significantly when sodium content in a beverage is relatively high (100 mmol sodium per liter fluid).[212] Although plasma potassium concentrations also tend to decline with intense exercise, in most cases the dietary intake of potassium (assuming it is appropriate) is sufficient for maintaining adequate potassium levels.[210] On the other hand, some people do suggest that including potassium in beverages postexercise may help rehydration by maintaining water in the intracellular space.[212]

The oral rehydration solution (ORS) recommended by the World Health Organization for the treatment of acute diarrhea has a sodium content of 60 to 90 mmol/L. However, the sodium content of most sports drinks is in the range of 10 to 25 mmol/L and in some cases is even lower. Most commonly consumed soft drinks contain no sodium and therefore are likely to be less effective at rehydration. These beverages are also less likely to stimulate fluid consumption than sodium-containing beverages. It appears, however, that high sodium beverages are often found to be unpalatable, resulting in reduced consumption. One possible solution might be to add a small amount of carbohydrate to the beverage, which may improve the rate of intestinal uptake of sodium and water and will improve palatability.[212]

Electron Transport System (ETS) The electron transport system accounts for the vast majority of adenosine triphosphate (ATP) production in the body. A comprehensive description of the ETS and each of its components is beyond the scope of this book. Briefly, the role of the "chain" of molecules in the ETS is to shuttle electrons from one component in the inner mitochondrial membrane to another via a series of oxidatio–reduction reactions with the ultimate production of ATP from adinosine diphosphate (ADP) as well as water. This process has been termed oxidative phosphorylation. Coenzyme forms of niacin and riboflavin are particularly instrumental in the process, since they serve as the initial electron donors. These molecules are produced in the metabolism of macronutrients by several metabolic pathways including glycolysis, beta-oxidation, and Krebs cycle.

Energy is often defined as the capacity to do work. Several forms of energy are extremely important in human physiology and biochemistry. These forms include chemical energy, such as ATP and macronutrients from food; mechanical energy, such as that which occurs with movement during a muscle contraction; heat, which is produced as a byproduct of metabolism and maintains thermoregulation; and electrical impulses.

Energy balance When an individual is in energy balance, dietary energy consumed is equal to energy expended. If energy intake exceeds energy expenditure, the net gain in energy will result in weight gain. On the other hand, if energy expenditure exceeds intake, weight loss will ensue.

Enzyme An enzyme is a protein that serves as a catalyst for a chemical reaction. In metabolism, most chemical reactions are reversible and require the enzyme for both directions of the reactions.

EPA *See* **Eicosapentaenoic acid**

Ephedra The term ephedra is used to refer to the herb "Ephedra sinica," which is also known as "ma huang." The ingredient of ephedra that has received the most attention with relation to athletic performance is ephedrine. See the entry on ephedrine for more information on its potential use as an ergogenic aid.

Ephedrine is a stimulant that can be obtained from the herb ma huang also known as Ephedra sinica. The Food and Drug Administration (FDA) has prohibited the sale of dietary supplements containing ephedrine alkaloids and has recommended that Americans discontinue its use. Those supplements were previously marketed for a variety of reasons, but especially as a way to increase energy expenditure and weight loss. As reviewed by Williams, while several studies have not detected positive effects on athletic performance, a few have, particularly when ephedrine was combined with caffeine.[214] Since the FDA has concluded that ephedrine-containing supplements pose an unreasonable health risk, particularly with regard to the heart, ephedrine can not be recommended as an ergogenic aid.

Epinephrine is a catecholamine also known as adrenaline that is produced in the adrenal glands from the metabolism of tyrosine. Classically speaking, epinephrine is known for its association with the fight or flight response. Release of epinephrine in situations of stress, such as exercise, shifts metabolism in ways that allow for the production of energy to drive chemical reactions. For example, initiation of exercise results in the release of epinephrine from the adrenal glands, which promotes mobilization of triglyceride-bound fatty acids stored within adipose tissue.

Ergogenic aid An ergogenic aid is a device, substance, or technique that can be used to increase athletic performance. Specifically, the word's root "ergo" refers to "work" and "genic" means "producing"; thus, an ergogenic aid allows for the production of work. Ergogenic aids have been classified into many broad categories including nutritional, pharmacological, physiological, psychological, and biomechanical aids. Much of this book describes potential nutritional ergogenic aids, which are foods, nutrients, or dietary supplements that can improve performance. Pharmacological aids are those that are drug-related, such as steroids. Caffeine is a pharmacological ergogenic aid that can also be considered nutritional since it can be found in foods such as coffee, tea, and soft drinks. Physiological aids can often be classified as nutritional or pharmacological as well and are those substances that alter the body's physiology in a manner favorable for athletic performance. Another example of a physiological ergogenic aid is the process of blood doping, in which blood is drawn at intervals for several weeks, then the red blood cells are reinfused prior to competition to increase the blood's oxygen-carrying capacity. Psychological ergogenic aids include techniques such as imaging, in which the athlete mentally goes through the steps of his or her performance prior to beginning the competition or event. Biomechanical ergogenic aids are those that provide an advantage in movement. Commonly cited examples include light-weight shoes for runners and strong, flexible poles for pole-vaulting.

Ergogenic prospect The term "ergogenic aid" can be extremely misleading. One often perceives a compound called an ergogenic aid as a product that is sure to improve athletic performance. In reality, this term is used to describe both effective and ineffective supplements marketed to improve performance. More accurate terminology for unproven products is needed to avoid confusion for athletes, coaches, athletic trainers, and others. The term ergogenic aid should be reserved for devices, substances, or techniques for which there is a general consensus regarding efficacy of the product to improve athletic performance. A term that more accurately reflects the dubious nature of unproven products is "ergogenic prospect."[215] This term neither suggests that a product is effective nor does it suggest that it is ineffective, instead it describes a product for which there is inadequate high quality scientific evidence to suggest that the product is truly ergogenic. It can also be used when referring to the use of a known ergogenic aid for specific purposes for which there is an absence of research demonstrating positive effects. For example, creatine is typically regarded as a true ergogenic aid for repetitive high intensity exercise bouts. However, it is not considered effective in improving endurance; thus, for repetitive sprints it may accurately be called an ergogenic aid, but for endurance events it should be considered an ergogenic prospect.

Ergolytic The term ergolytic was coined to mean the opposite of ergogenic. A device, substance, or technique that hinders performance is considered ergolytic.

Essential amino acid An essential amino acid is required in the diet of humans because we lack the ability to produce adequate amounts to meet our needs for normal growth, development, and maintenance. A term that is often used interchangeably with essential is "indispensable," since we cannot do without it. Table A.1 in the entry for amino acids provides a list of all the essential amino acids. Each essential amino acid is described in more detail in separate entries.

Essential fatty acid An essential fatty acid is required in the diet of humans because we lack the ability to produce them ourselves. Linoleate and alpha-linolenate are the only essential fatty acids for humans. They are essential because we lack the delta-12 and delta-15 desaturase enzymes that are required to insert the double bonds needed in the final steps of the synthesis of these fatty acids. Dietary deficiency produces dermatitis, decreased growth or weight loss, organ dysfunction, and abnormal reproductive status. Separate entries for the essential fatty acids are provided.

Essential nutrient An essential nutrient is required in the diet of humans because we lack the ability to produce adequate amounts to meet our needs for normal growth, development, and maintenance.

Estimated Average Requirement (EAR) The Estimated Average Requirement (EAR) is one of four possible Dietary Reference Intake (DRI) values established by the Food and Nutrition Board of the National

Academy of Sciences. The EAR is a value for a nutrient that reflects the average need of individuals of a particular age range and gender. This value can be used to assess nutrient needs or adequacy of a group on the whole. The Recommended Dietary Allowance (RDA) or Adequate Intake (AI) for a particular nutrient is calculated as two standard deviations above the EAR.

Estrogen is a steroid hormone ultimately synthesized from cholesterol. It is especially important for female reproduction and the development of typical female characteristics. The entry for the female athlete triad describes a situation when inadequate estrogen production puts athletes at a high risk for bone loss.

Ethanol *See* **Alcohol**

Extracellular water Water that is found outside of the cell is referred to as extracellular water. This fluid includes the intravascular water that is not within the cells, lymph fluids, and water within tissues, but between the cells. Extracellular water accounts for approximately 45% of the body's total water content.

F

Facilitated diffusion is similar to diffusion in that a substance (such as a solute in a solution) moves from an area of high concentration to an area of low concentration. However, with facilitated diffusion, the movement occurs across a membrane by the assistance of a carrier molecule. Without the carrier, diffusion of that substance would not occur.

Fasting simply means abstaining from consumption of food for a period of time such as during sleep. A typical period of time for a fast for assessing nutritional status is 12 hours; however, fasts can be established for longer or shorter periods.

Fast-twitch muscle fiber Muscle fibers that have a high contractile speed are considered fast-twitch and are also known as type II fibers. Type II differ from type I fibers, which are considered slow-twitch. Type II fibers are typically classified based on their preferred manner of energy utilization. For example, type IIa fibers, also known as fast-twitch red muscle fibers, produce energy via both the aerobic and anaerobic metabolism of glucose. These fibers differ from type IIb fibers, also known as fast-twitch white fibers, which produce energy primarily via aerobic metabolism. Due to their tendency to produce energy anaerobically, these fibers are often called fast-glycolytic (FG) fibers, while type IIa fibers are called fast-oxidative glycolytic (FOG) fibers.

Fat loading The process of fat loading derives its name from the term carbohydrate loading, a technique of consuming a very high carbohydrate diet in the days leading up to competition. Fat loading techniques that have been the topic of a significant amount of scientific research vary from carbohydrate loading in two major ways. One is that the diet is very high in fat instead of carbohydrate and the other is that a longer-term approach of eating the modified diet is required. Another difference is that carbohydrate loading is predicated on the notion of maximizing stores of carbohydrate energy within the body, while the metabolic goal of fat loading is to enhance the body's ability to utilize fat for energy during competition, thereby sparing the stored carbohydrate energy and prolonging endurance.

Results of studies assessing the efficacy of fat loading for improving endurance performance have been equivocal and some of the research that supports an enhancement has been highly criticized for design flaws. Since several studies have demonstrated that a high-carbohydrate diet helps to maintain glycogen stores,[104] most researchers feel that it is counterintuitive to believe that fat loading can enhance performance. In actuality, several researchers have detected either no difference[216] in performance of athletes adapted to high-fat vs. high-carbohydrate diets for up to several weeks or enhancement by fat adaptation,[217–219] and fewer have detected adverse effects from a fat-rich diet.[220]

Overall, with equivocal data and the risk of low muscle glycogen content while consuming a high-fat diet, it is prudent to continue to recommend that most athletes consume a nutrient-dense lower fat diet until more conclusive data are available to suggest that fat loading is effective. Given the possibility that adaptation to a high-fat diet may minimize glycogen utilization during exercise, more studies are needed to corroborate the findings of Lambert et al., which suggest that adaptation to a diet rich in fats followed by short-term high carbohydrate intake in the days prior to competition can optimize endurance.[221] It is also important to note that the adverse effects of a diet rich in fat, even primarily saturated fat, are blunted in athletes.[222,223] This research should not serve as a "license to eat" for athletes, however, since many other risk factors for chronic diseases have not been evaluated in athletes consuming a diet rich in saturated fatty acids. With data mounting in favor of potential ergogenic benefits of a higher fat diet, athletes who do not have body weight control issues may wish to assess their exercise response to consuming a diet rich in "healthy" fats, particularly when followed by short-term carbohydrate loading.

Fat-soluble vitamins Vitamins that dissolve in organic solvents (such as chloroform, etc.) are considered fat-soluble vitamins and include vitamins A, D, E, and K. In general fat-soluble vitamins are absorbed via the lymphatic system along with other fat-soluble nutrients. Within the bloodstream, fat-soluble vitamins must be transported as complexes bound to lipoproteins or specific transport proteins. Fat-soluble vitamins can be stored within lipid-rich tissues, such as adipose and the liver. Clinical deficiency of any of the fat-soluble vitamins is likely to impair athletic performance; however, research supporting a benefit for their supplementation to improve performance is scant at best. Separate entries are provided for each of the fat-soluble vitamins as well as beta-carotene, a precursor for vitamin A.

Fatigue can be defined as either emotional or physical tiredness. A primary goal of sports nutrition is to prevent fatigue during training or competition, in order to maximize fitness and athletic peformance. Fatigue can be produced by a variety of mechanisms and has the potential to hinder performance by many means. For example, in skill sports such as tennis, fatigue may reduce the athlete's ability to accurately strike the ball.[224] Another fatigue-induced hindrance to performance is a decrease in physical work capacity, which could affect performance in most sports.

Fatigue can be produced either centrally or peripherally. Central fatigue involves fatigue as sensed by the central nervous system. Peripheral fatigue is related to noncentral components such as the muscle or organ systems. In endurance exercise a primary cause of peripheral fatigue is an inadequate fuel supply. Much of sports nutrition surrounds foods, nutrients, supplements, or dietary techniques designed to maximize fuel supply and utilization. For more information regarding central fatigue, see the entry on central fatigue theory.

Fats (also known as lipids) are characterized by their ability to dissolve in organic solvents (such as choloroform, etc.). When speaking specifically about dietary fat, most nutritionists are referring to triglycerides, the specific class of lipids that comprise the vast majority (>95%) of lipids in the diet. Other lipids in the diet or the body include fatty acids, monoglycerides, diglycerides, phospholipids, sterols, some vitamins, lipoproteins, glycolipids, and other important molecules. Separate entries are provided for many of these lipids. Lipids in general possess a large array of functions, which include providing energy, serving as major structural components to cells, and participating in important biochemical processes.

Fatty acids are lipid molecules characterized by a hydrocarbon chain bound to a carboxylic acid group (Figure F.1). Fatty acids are often referred to as acyl groups in biochemistry. Fatty acids vary in many ways, structurally, nutritionally, and biochemically, which has led to many classifications for fatty acids as well as fats (triglycerides) rich in particular classes of fatty acids.

One classification is based on the length of the fatty acid, as determined by the number of carbon atoms of the hydrocarbon chain. Typically, fatty acids have an even number of carbons, although some

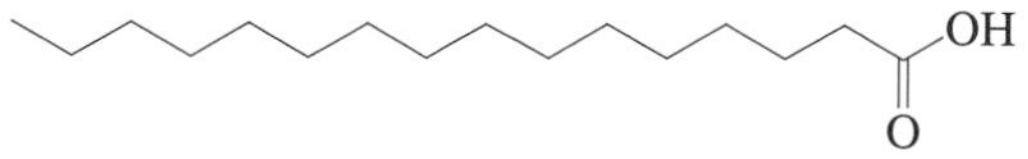

fatty acid (palmitic acid)

FIGURE F.1

less common fatty acids have an odd number. Short-chain fatty acids include molecules with 2 to 4 carbons. Medium-chain fatty acids are usually classified as those possessing 6 to 10 carbons, and long-chain fatty acids have 12 or more carbons. The majority of fatty acids in the human diet are long-chain fatty acids. In general, most long-chain saturated fatty acids come from animal foods, coconut oil, palm oil, and palm kernel oil. Monounsaturated fatty acids are found in high levels in canola oil, olives and olive oil, avocados, and several other plant foods and oils. Fish, nuts, seeds, and many other vegetable oils tend to be rich in polyunsaturated fatty acids. Although we obtain small amounts of short- and medium-chain fatty acids from foods such as dairy products and coconut oil, relatively little quantities of these fatty acids are found in a natural diet. Medium-chain fatty acids, produced primarily from the fractionation of coconut oil, are commonly used in dietary supplements and formulas for medical nutrition therapy.

Fatty acids are also commonly classified based on their degree of saturation with hydrogen atoms, which is determined by the absence or presence of double bonds between carbon atoms. Saturated fatty acids have no double bonds and are therefore "saturated" with hydrogen ions. Unsaturated fatty acids have at least one double bond. Those fatty acids with a single double bond are called monounsaturated fatty acids (MUFAs), while those that have more than one double bond are called polyunsaturated fatty acids (PUFAs).

Unsaturated fatty acids can be further classified based on the structure of the molecules around the double bond as well as the position of the double bond within the hydrocarbon chain. Since carbon molecules require four bonds, the carbons linked by a double bond have only a single hydrogen bound to each of them. If the hydrogen molecules on the double bonded carbons are oriented on the same side of the hydrocarbon chain, the bond is considered to have a *cis* configuration. These hydrogen molecules interact to produce what has been called a bend in the hydrocarbon chain. Fatty acids with a *trans* configuration have hydrogen atoms oriented across from one another, which allows the hydrocarbon to take on what is considered a straighter structure. These differences in structure produce vastly different effects on metabolism.

The position of the double bond or bonds on the hydrocarbon chain is also important for determining the metabolism of unsaturated fatty acids. The classification most commonly used by nutritionists is the omega classification, which is determined by the position of the first double bond when counting from the hydrocarbon end. Fatty acids

TABLE F.1
Characteristics of Common Fatty Acids

Name	Chain Length	Double Bonds	Omega Class
SCFAs			
Acetate	2	0	NA
Propionate	3	0	NA
Butyrate	4	0	NA
MCFAs			
Caproate	6	0	NA
Caprylate	8	0	NA
Caprate	10	0	NA
LCFAs			
Laurate*	12	0	NA
Myristate	14	0	NA
Palmitate	16	0	NA
Stearate	18	0	NA
Oleate	18	1	9
Linoleate	18	2	6
α-Linolenate	18	3	3
γ-Linolenate	18	3	6
Arachindonate	20	4	6
Eicospentaenoate	20	5	3
Docosahexaenoate	22	6	3

* Sometimes classified as a medium-chain fatty acid.

with the first double bond on the third carbon are called omega-3 fatty acids, those with the first double bond on the number 6 carbon are called omega-6 fatty acids, and so on. While the amount of energy produced from catabolism of fatty acids is similar regardless of its omega classification, positions of double bonds are critical for determining other functions of fatty acids. Table F.1 provides a summary of many fatty acids along with information regarding their structure and dietary sources.

Two fatty acids are also classified as essential fatty acids, linoleic acid and alpha-linolenic acid (the omega-3 form of linolenic acid), since they are required in the human diet. Some details of their essentialities are described in the entry for essential fatty acids.

Fatty acids are extremely important to athletes for normal biochemistry as well as for the production of energy. Metabolism of fatty acids during exercise is described in the entry for free fatty acids. Many specific fatty acids and fatty acids within particular classifications have been studied for their potential ergogenic benefits; thus, where appropriate, further information for some fats and fatty acids are provided in their respective entries.

FDA *See* **Food and Drug Administration**

Female athlete triad The number of girls participating in sports has increased tremendously in the past three decades. However, in recent years a new concern has arisen with the development of the female athlete triad, or the "Triad." [225,226] The Triad is a serious syndrome that consists of disordered eating, amenorrhea, and osteoporosis. The Triad was initially thought to occur in elite athletes alone; however, it was later discovered that it can also occur in physically active women of all ages from all varieties of sports.[203] Pressure to achieve and maintain a particular body weight or body shape might put the female athlete at risk for developing disordered eating behaviors. Those behaviors usually include food restriction and pathogenic weight control behaviors that might lead to menstrual dysfunction and to a subsequent decrease in bone mineral density. Without treatment, the bone loss could eventually result in osteoporosis. Alone or in combination, the disorders of the Triad can negatively affect health and impair athletic performance. When all three components of the Triad appear together it can result in even more serious problems and may even become life threatening.[225]

Relatively few studies have examined the prevalence of the Triad among female athletes. However, according to existing data the prevalence of those at risk might be as high as 62% in certain sports.[227] According to the American College of Sports Medicine, girls and women who participate in sports that emphasize low body weight and lean appearance, such as distance running, skiing, and cycling; require revealing more body, such as gymnastics, swimming, diving, and cheerleading; require subjective ratings, such as gymnastics, figure skating, and aerobics; and have weight categories, such as wrestling and rowing, are at the greatest risk for developing one or more of the components of the Triad.[203]

Disordered eating can be defined as a wide spectrum of harmful and often ineffective eating behaviors used in an attempt to lose weight or achieve a lean appearance.[203] The spectrum of disordered eating behaviors ranges from mild to severe. The term disordered eating is often used to describe many abnormal eating behaviors, which at their extreme include anorexia nervosa and bulimia nervosa. The majority of athletes are more likely to experience disordered eating behaviors at subclinical levels than to exhibit a true eating disorder, since many do not meet the diagnostic criteria for either anorexia nervosa or bulimia nervosa.[227]

There are serious medical consequences as a result of eating disorders, which include depleted glycogen stores, decreased lean body mass, chronic fatigue, micronutrient deficiencies, dehydration, anemia, electrolyte and acid-base imbalances, hypoglycemia, gastrointestinal disorders, parotid gland enlargement, cardiac arrhythmia, amenorrhea, decreased bone density, and erosion of tooth enamel. There are also many psychological problems that often accompany disordered eating behaviors, including decreased self-esteem, anxiety, depression, and death from suicide or cardiac arrhythmia.[203,225] In addition to the risk of developing severe health complications, disordered eating behaviors might impair athletic and work performance, and increase the risk of injury. Decreased caloric intake, and resulting fluid and electrolyte imbalances, can produce decreased endurance, strength, reaction time, speed, and ability to concentrate.[227]

Amenorrhea is usually defined as the absence of three or more consecutive menstrual cycles. Primary amenorrhea or delayed menarche is the absence of menstruation by age 16 in a girl with secondary sex characteristics. Secondary amenorrhea is the absence of three or more consecutive menstrual cycles after menarche.[225] Menstrual dysfunction is common in adolescents who are involved in intensive athletic activity or who limit their nutritional intake excessively.[228] Sometimes the menstrual dysfunction occurs with the complete cessation of menstruation and sometimes with periods of oligomenorrhea. Oligomenorrhea is defined as a menstrual cycle lasting more than 36 days.[225]

Among females in the general population, the prevalence of amenorrhea is 2 to 5%, while among female athletes the prevalence ranges between 3 to 66%. The large range is a result of different definitions of amenorrhea and different study populations.[229] Risk factors for the development of athletic amenorrhea include low energy intake, low protein intake, low body weight, low body fat, and intense training. There is no exact threshold of body weight, body fat percentage, or amount of training that will universally initiate the development of amenorrhea in an athlete.[227]

Amenorrhea was once considered a relatively benign and "normal" response to physical training. However, today professionals recognize menstrual dysfunction as a serious medical condition. Athletic amenorrhea is a severe problem because of the potential catastrophic skeletal effect and the risk of decreased bone density and premature osteoporosis that is associated with it.[225] The bone mineral loss seen in women athletes who have had amenorrhea for more than 6 months resembles that observed in women after menopause.[226]

The loss of estrogen due to menstrual disturbances has major effects on bone. Calcium homeostasis becomes less efficient, resulting in an increased calcium intake from the bones, which is necessary to maintain calcium balance. Secondly, an estrogen deficiency permits osteoclasts to resorb bone with greater efficiency.[227] The decreased bone mineral density can often produce multiple or recurring stress fractures.[225] Research during the past 10 years has shown that the premature osteoporosis in women with amenorrhea is partially irreversible despite resumption of menses, estrogen replacement, or calcium supplementation.[227]

Osteoporosis affects 25 million individuals in the U.S. and causes 1.5 million fractures each year.[227] Approximately 60 to 70% of peak bone mass in women is acquired before the age of 20. Peak bone mineral density (BMD) is usually achieved between the ages of 18 to 25 years in women,[230] although recent research has suggested that BMD may peak even sooner at some bone sites.[231] It is imperative that young women maximize their peak BMD to avoid osteoporosis later in life. If bone loss is secondary to amenorrhea, restoration of normal menses may inhibit the rate of further bone loss, but the bone is not likely to be replaced. Despite high-intensity exercise that increases BMD, athletes with amenorrhea have significantly lower whole-body BMD than athletes without amenorrhea or nonathletes.[225]

Efforts to prevent the development of disordered eating behaviors in female athletes are critical, yet little is known regarding how to accomplish this. Most practitioners in this area suggest that a key is to avoid promoting behaviors that can lead to an eating disorder and ultimately the female athlete triad.

FFA *See* Free fatty acids

Fiber is a group of nondigestible polysachharides found in plant foods as well as lignin, which is primarily associated with the structural components of plants. Although fibers are not digestible by enzymes of the human intestinal tract, colonic bacteria possess the ability to ferment some fiber, not lignin, thereby producing short-chain fatty acids that can be absorbed by the colonic epithelium and provide some energy to the body. Therefore, while the term nondigestible is accurate regarding human digestion, some fiber digestion does occur within the human body.

Fibers are usually classified as those that are soluble in water and those that are insoluble in water. Water-soluble fibers that are common in the diet include pectins, gums, mucilages, algal polysaccharides, beta-glucans, pysllium, resistant starches, and inulin. Water insoluble fibers include cellulose, some hemicelluloses, and lignin.

The potential impact of fiber on exercise performance has not been directly studied. Most practitioners recommend that the typical diet of an athlete contain similar amounts of fiber to those recommended for the general population (usually about 20 to 35 grams per day). However, for meals consumed prior to or during competition, most recommend foods low in fiber to avoid gastrointestinal discomfort, which may negatively impact performance.

Actual research does not necessarily support the notion that moderate amounts of fiber will produce adverse effects for competition. In fact, as described in the entry on the glycemic index, consumption of some fiber-containing foods has produced a lower preexercise glycemic response and improvements in performance. Other studies have not demonstrated improvements in performance but report no decreases in performance, either. Until solid research for recommendations is available, the amount of fiber that an athlete should consume before competition depends on how well the athlete can tolerate foods that contain fiber and must be determined on a case-by-case basis.

Fluids *See* **Hydration status**

Fluorine is a micromineral most often considered in its fluoride form as an ingredient in toothpastes and as an additive in drinking water. Although drinking water provides the majority of fluoride in the diets of most individuals, it is also found in seafood, particularly when the bones are eaten. Smaller amounts are found in a variety of foods from each of the food groups. Fluoride is particularly important for the production of strong bones and teeth. No roles for fluorine supplementation to enhance performance have been established.

Folacin *See* **Folic acid**

Folate *See* **Folic acid**

Folic acid (see Figure F.2), sometimes referred to as folate or folacin, is a water-soluble vitamin found in green leafy vegetables, whole grains, legumes, and many fruits. Folic acid exists in many interconverted forms and functions in the synthesis of DNA, which makes it extremely important for normal cell division. It is perhaps best known for the prevention of neural tube defects in infants when consumed at adequate levels by pregnant women. Deficiency of folic acid produces abnormally large and immature red blood cells that are poorly functioning; therefore, dietary deficiency is one of several causes of megaloblastic anemia. Like other anemias, megaloblastic anemia can limit the physical work capacity of an individual.

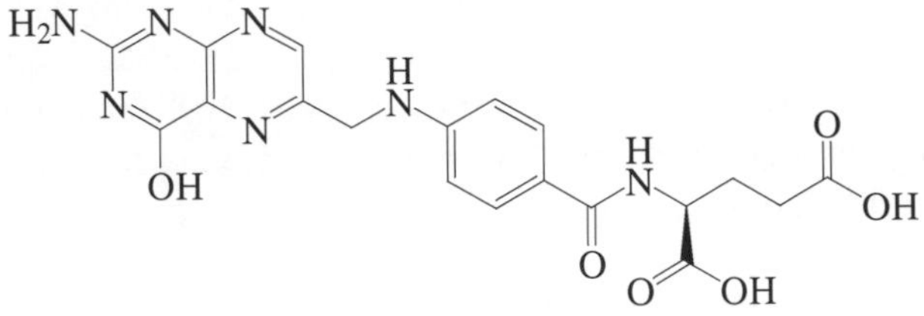

folic acid

FIGURE F.2

Adequate folic acid is critical for optimal performance. In one study, malnourished, anemic children were dewormed and then provided a supplement of folic acid and iron for 2 months.[232] At the end of the time period, measures of physical work capacity were tremendously increased. However, this study should not be used to suggest that folic acid will improve performance in well-nourished athletes, but the data rather suggest that folic acid or iron deficiency will prevent optimal performance. In fact, no data are available to support that folic acid supplements can enhance performance in healthy individuals. Studies in which folic acid was included as part of a multivitamin supplement also failed to demonstrate performance enhancement.[233,234]

Food and Drug Administration (FDA) The Food and Drug Administration is a component of the United States Department of Health and Human Services. The scope of areas regulated by the FDA are vast and include food (including dietary supplements), drugs, medical devices, biologics (such as vaccines, blood products, etc.), animal feed and drugs for both livestock and pets, cosmetics, radiation-emitting products, and combination products. The FDA's Center for Food Safety and Applied Nutrition (CFSAN) is the hub for regulatory activities regarding food, nutrition, and dietary supplements.

Food Guide Pyramid The Food Guide Pyramid provides a specific set of recommendations for consuming an adequate diet without excess intake of energy, fat, saturated fat, cholesterol, added sugars, sodium, and alcohol. The Pyramid was developed as a practical representation of food selection for the *Dietary Guidelines for Americans*, which is described in the entry on dietary recommendations for athletes. Although more specific than the basic dietary guidelines, a major strength of the Pyramid is that it allows the user a high degree of freedom to make selections that fit his or her personal beliefs, tastes, financial status, and other factors affecting dietary intake. The Pyramid can be viewed and downloaded at the Web site for the Food and

Nutrition Information Center of the National Library of Medicine (www.nal.usda.gov/fnic/).

Free fatty acids (FFA) are lipid molecules characterized by a hydrocarbon chain bound to a carboxylic acid group. Free fatty acids are generally classified as those fatty acids found in the bloodstream that are not bound to a glycerol molecule (as in triglycerides, phospholipids, and so forth), to cholesterol in the formation of cholesterol esters, or as a component of other molecules. The term free fatty acid, however, is a misnomer, since as lipid soluble molecules, they cannot be found in the free form in an aqueous environment. In fact, free fatty acids are typically found in the bloodstream bound to albumin.

F

During exercise, free fatty acids are mobilized into the bloodstream from triglyceride molecules stored in adipose tissue in response to the action of hormone sensitive lipase. As the fatty acids reach the circulation, they are rapidly bound to albumin and transported through the circulatory system. Tissues that require fatty acids for energy production (for example, skeletal muscle, etc.) take up the fatty acid. As it enters the cell, the fatty acid is bound to a coenzyme A molecule at the expense of adenosine triphosphate (ATP). From within the cell, the fatty acids are translocated to the mitochondria via the functions of carnitine and the enzyme carnitine translocase. During this process, the coenzyme A molecule is left behind in the cytosol of the cell, but the fatty acid is bound to another coenzyme A molecule within the mitochondria. Fatty acids bound to coenzyme A molecules are referred to as fatty acyl CoA molecules. These compounds are considered the "activated" form of a fatty acid within the mitochondria. They can then be oxidized via beta-oxidation, which produces acetyl CoA, $NADH + H^+$, and $FADH_2$ molecules. Acetyl CoA can enter Krebs cycle, which produces additional $NADH + H^+$ and $FADH_2$ molecules as well as guanosine triphosphate (GTP), which is a high-energy molecule similar to ATP. The $NADH + H^+$ and $FADH_2$ molecules produced via beta-oxidation and Krebs cycle initiate oxidative phosphorylation via the electron transport system to produce ATP.

Free radicals are atoms or molecules with at least one unpaired electron. Unpaired electrons in the orbitals of atoms produce highly reactive species that promote oxidative damage. Lipid peroxide, superoxide, hydroxyl, and hydroperoxyl radicals are commonly produced in metabolism. Nitric oxide and nitrogen dioxide are nitrogen-containing free radicals. Other reactive molecules include singlet oxygen, hydrogen peroxide, and many others.

Free radicals can oxidize many vital chemicals in the body including DNA, proteins, and polyunsaturated fatty acids. Oxidation of these constituents can produce a variety of damaging effects that can influence the risk for chronic diseases such as cancer, heart disease, and others. Formation of free radicals and their subsequent oxidation of these molecules is a natural process; however, the body and diet provide many antioxidant defenses that can protect the molecules from excess damage. See the entry for antioxidants for a description of the roles of antioxidants in preventing oxidative damage during exercise.

Fructose (Figure F.3) is a 6-carbon monosaccharide (a hexose) primarily found in food in either its simple form or bound to glucose as part of the disaccharide sucrose. Foods rich in this monosaccharide itself include many fruits and honey, although much of the fructose in the diet is consumed in foods such as soft drinks, sports drinks, baked goods, and

fructose

FIGURE F.3

so forth, that are sweetened with high fructose corn syrup. Since one-half of the sucrose molecule is fructose, foods rich in sucrose also provide much of the fructose in the diet.

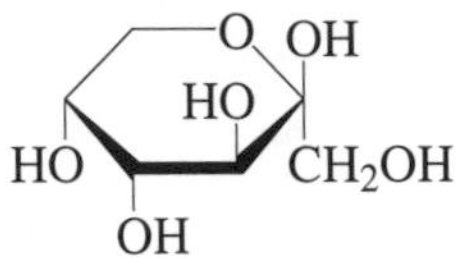

Unlike the other primary monosaccharides found in our diet, glucose and galactose, fructose is absorbed by a facilitated diffusion process. This mechanism is saturable, meaning that the rate of fructose absorption is limited, which produces absorption at a slower rate. Because it is absorbed more slowly than other carbohydrates, particularly when fed in the absence of other carbohydrates, it produces a lower glycemic response, which in turn produces a lower insulinemic response. This slower absorption has been considered a cause for concern for athletes, since large amounts of fructose residing in the gut for an extended period of time can produce gastrointestinal distress including cramping and diarrhea. However, as described in the glycemic index entry, foods producing a lower glycemic response may be beneficial for performance as preexercise feedings when compared to those that produce a higher glycemic response.

When consumed during exercise, there are no reported benefits of pure fructose feedings in comparison to other carbohydrates. Alternatively, since large amounts of fructose can produce symptoms of gastrointestinal distress, feedings high in fructose during exercise are often discouraged.

G

Galactose (Figure G.1) is a 6-carbon monosaccharide (a hexose) found in the diet primarily as part of the disaccharide lactose. Other foods containing galactose include peas, lentils, some legumes, organ meats, cereals, and some fruits and vegetables. In the past few years, sports foods providing galactose have gained in popularity, yet little research is available to support a benefit for performance in comparison to other carbohydrates. One study has determined that feeding galactose 45 minutes prior to cycling exercise produces a lower glycemic and insulinemic response in comparison to glucose.[235] However, no difference in cycling performance was detected in that study. Another study demonstrated that galactose oxidation during 2 hours of exercise is approximately half that of glucose.[236]

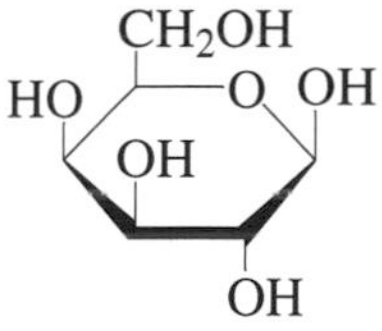

galactose

FIGURE G.1

Garcinia cambogia The herb *Garcinia cambogia* is a very small purple fruit native to India and Southeast Asia. This herb has been a popular weight loss aid due to its richness in a substance called hydroxycitric acid, or HCA, which is closely related to the citric acid found in grapefruits and oranges and has been marketed for improving body composition. Some extremely limited research has demonstrated that supplementing with *Garcinia cambogia* flavonoids decreased serum concentrations of total cholesterol, triglycerides, and the hormone leptin[237,238]; however, evidence is not able to support a direct role in weight loss or decreased body fat.

Gastric emptying The rate of gastric (stomach) emptying after consumption of foods and beverages has potentially important influences with regard to athletic performance. Dietary (or nondietary) factors that slow the rate of gastric emptying can limit fuel availability for exercise, thus adversely impacting performance. Many have suggested that a slower rate of gastric emptying could produce gastrointestinal discomfort, which may hinder athletic performance, and would likely reduce the rate of water absorption increasing risk for dehydration-related performance impairment. Conversely, a meted release of food from the stomach may produce a steadier flow of nutrients, such as glucose, into the bloodstream. Some have suggested that this may produce lower glycemic and insulinemic responses, which may result in performance benefits from preexercise feedings.

Generally recognized as safe (GRAS) Any additive approved for use in foods must be generally recognized as safe as determined by the Food and Drug Administration (FDA).

Ginkgo biloba Extracts of ginkgo biloba have antioxidant properties similar to those of many other compounds including green tea. Studies of potential ergogenic effects do not appear to be available. In limited research, however, ginkgo has been demonstrated to decrease lipid peroxidation *in vitro*.[239] Currently, ginkgo biloba show no recognized alterations in metabolism that could be implicated in enhanced exercise performance.

Ginseng refers to a group of plants or plant extracts from the Araliaceae family. There are three different herbs commonly called ginseng: Asian or Korean ginseng (Panax ginseng), American ginseng (Panax quinquefolius), and Siberian ginseng (Eleutherococcus senticosus). Ginsenosides are considered the active ingredients in this family. While many health-related benefits of ginseng have been claimed, few have been substantiated by well-conducted research. The claims used by those who market ginseng to athletes include an ability to enhance endurance exercise performance and to reduce fatigue in general. In 2000, a review of research surrounding this topic concluded that there is a lack of evidence supporting an ergogenic effect of ginseng for humans.[240]

Panax ginseng has shown some promise as a mild ergogenic aid, but published evidence remains incomplete and contradictory, and most of the research conducted has been poorly controlled. A few well-controlled studies have suggested that ergogenic effects may occur, and usually only with supplements of higher doses using standardized extracts with longer supplementation durations.[241] Bucci provided a general recommendation for the use of standardized Panax ginseng for at least 8 weeks at a dose of at least 200 mg/day.[241] However, recent well-designed research has failed to demonstrate positive effects of ginseng under these conditions.[242,243]

Although excess use of ginseng may produce ginseng abuse syndrome, this effect is not common. The symptoms of ginseng abuse syndrome include high blood pressure, nervousness, and sleeplessness.[244] However, reports of this syndrome have been somewhat discredited as a result of poorly controlled research. It has been noted that the subjects reporting these symptoms consumed extremely large amounts of ginseng (up to 15 g per day), with many consuming concomitantly large levels of caffeine. Most of the symptoms of ginseng abuse syndrome are also associated with consumption of large amounts of caffeine.[244]

A health care provider should be consulted for those athletes who wish to supplement with Asian ginseng in cases of acute illness, hypertension, and when using large amounts of stimulants like caffeine-containing beverages. In addition, athletes taking phenelzine, warfarin, or zidovidin should consult with a health care provider before using ginseng.[244]

Overall, of the studies considered well designed, the majority have not produced positive effects. Until conclusive evidence is available, recommending these supplements for athletes is not warranted.

Glucagon is a peptide hormone synthesized in the alpha cells of the pancreas. A primary function of glucagon is in the regulation of blood glucose, in which it most notably raises blood glucose by simulating gluconeogenesis and glycogenolysis. Upon the initiation of exercise, glucagon production and secretion is enhanced to provide glucose to working muscles.

Glucomannan is a component of konjac root, and has a chemical structure similar to that of galactomannan from guar gum, which contains a polysaccharide chain of glucose and mannose. It has been claimed to reduce cholesterol, normalize blood sugar, relieve stress on the pancreas, depress blood sugar abnormalities, and support bowel health by binding toxic substances and eliminating them before they can be absorbed into the bloodstream. One study that examined the efficacy of glucomannan revealed that it produced significantly greater weight loss compared to a placebo.[245]

Gluconeogenesis As implied by the name, gluconeogenesis is a new beginning of glucose, or in other words, the production of glucose from noncarbohydrate substrates. Precursors of gluconeogenesis include glycerol, lactic acid, pyruvic acid, and many amino acids. The rate of gluconeogenesis is stimulated during exercise to provide more glucose to working muscles and other cells. The majority of gluconeogenesis occurs in the liver, since the cells of most tissues do not possess all of the needed enzymes.

Glucose (see Figure G.2) is a 6-carbon monosacharride (a hexose) found abundantly in many various forms in a wide array of foods. Free glucose is found in many fruits, honey, corn syrup, sports drinks, and a large assortment of other foods. Glucose is also a component of most other carbohydrates including, but not limited to, starch, sucrose, lactose, and maltose. Any foods rich in these nutrients ultimately provide the body with significant amounts of glucose. Furthermore, the other primary dietary monosaccharides fructose and galactose are ultimately converted to glucose or glucose derivatives after absorption. Since all carbohydrates can be converted into glucose, it is an extremely important nutrient physiologically. Glucose, however, can be made available for the body from more than just dietary carbohydrates. Many amino acids, glycerol, and pyruvic and lactic acids can be used to produce glucose through gluconeogenesis.

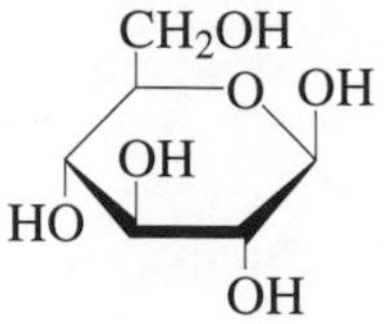

glucose

FIGURE G.2

G

Glucose serves as a primary fuel for the body and a highly preferred fuel for many cells including the central nervous system and red blood cells. The catabolism of glucose for energy in these cells and all others is called glycolysis. When athletes need to rapidly produce energy from glucose during very strenuous exercise that can last for only a short time, a large proportion of that glucose will be metabolized anaerobically to produce adenosine triphosphate (ATP) and the final product lactic acid. As the intensity of exercise decreases, aerobic glucose metabolism will predominate and although ATP will be produced less rapidly, the final product of glycolysis will be pyruvic acid, which can undergo further metabolism via the pyruvate dehydrogenase complex, followed by Krebs cycle and ultimately the electron transport system to produce additional ATP.

Glucose that is not needed for energy production can be stored until a time that it is needed. The storage form of glucose is glycogen, which is a very compact, highly-branched chain of glucose molecules linked together by glycosidic bonds. The majority of glycogen stored in the body is located in the muscles and liver. In times of energy need, glycogen is broken down via glycogenolysis to produce glucose or glucose derivatives. Glycogen within a muscle cell must be used for energy within that cell, since glycogenolysis continues only until the production of the molecule glucose-6-phosphate, which cannot escape the cell, but can enter the glycolytic pathway within the muscle cell for production of energy. Glycogen within liver cells can be broken down to free glucose molecules, because the liver produces an enzyme called glucose-6-phosphatase, which removes the phosphate molecule. Free glucose can leave the liver cell and travel via the circulation to tissues requiring energy production.

Another important function of glucose is the production of the 5-carbon sugar ribose. This is accomplished through a metabolic pathway called the hexosemonophosphate shunt or pentose pathway. Ribose is an important component of the base pairs of nucleic acids (i.e., DNA and RNA). The hexosemonophosphate shunt also produces NADPH, which is a coenzyme form of niacin that is involved in important functions including fatty acid synthesis.

Glucose polymers (or maltodextrins) are relatively short chains of glucose units linked by glycosidic bonds. Glucose polymers are produced by partial hydrolysis of starch molecules, which contain many more glucose units linked together. Although current evidence suggests that glucose polymers offer no advantage compared to other carbohydrates for exercise performance, they can theoretically be considered a preferred fuel for endurance athletes, since as larger particles they could provide more energy within fewer total molecules, which may provide an osmotic advantage over simpler carbohdyrates. Total molecules within a solution is the key for determining the osmotic load of a solution; thus, with fewer particles needed to produce a solution containing an equal or greater amount of energy, it is expected that more energy could be fed with less risk of interfering with fluid balance and production of gastrointestinal distress. Furthermore, this could allow for more rapid absorption of water; thus a solution containing glucose polymers may have a hydrating advantage over other beverages. Many sports foods containing glucose polymers will list those substances as maltodextrins on the food label.

Glutamic acid (Figure G.3), also known as glutamate, is a nonessential amino acid. Because it has two carboxylic acid groups, it is often classified along with aspartic acid as a diacidic amino acid. Glutamate is instrumentally involved in production of urea from the amino nitrogen of other amino acids. When glutamate accepts the ammonium ions produced in deamination of other amino acids, glutamine is formed. Glutamine is a primary donor of amino nitrogen for urea production as well.

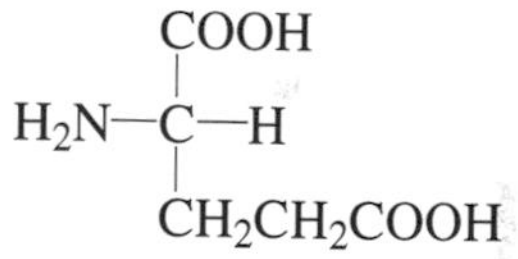

$$COOH$$
$$H_2N-C-H$$
$$CH_2CH_2COOH$$

glutamic acid

FIGURE G.3

Glutamate and its alpha-ketoacid counterpart (alpha-ketoglutarate) are vitally important as a donor and acceptor of amino groups, respectively, in transamination reactions, which are extremely important for production of nonessential amino acids and precursors for energy metabolism. When glutamate is deaminated, as in a transamination reaction, alpha-ketoglutarate is produced, which can be used for energy metabolism within Krebs cycle.

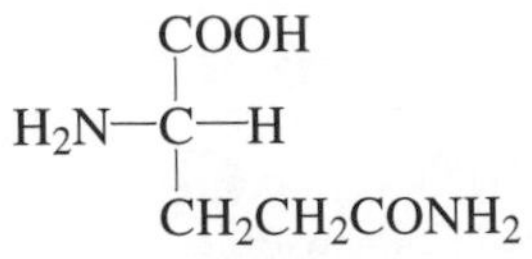

Glutamine (Figure G.4) is a nonessential amino acid. The functions of glutamine vary, but along with glutamate include serving as a donor of amino nitrogen for the production of urea. Glutamine is also an important energy source for intestinal cells and white blood cells. It has received considerable attention for its ergogenic potential and its involvement in the immune system for the prevention of illness in athletes.

$$COOH$$
$$H_2N-C-H$$
$$CH_2CH_2CONH_2$$

glutamine

FIGURE G.4

Glutamine has been studied as an ergogenic for both its endurance and anabolic potential. Research generally does not support a role for glutamine in enhancing strength or anabolism.[246] With regard to endurance, glutamine supplementation may improve the production of glycogen.[247] That research suggests high doses of glutamine improve the body's ability to store carbohydrates, but did not assess whether the effect can translate to improved endurance performance. Endurance performance was not improved in cyclists who consumed 0.03 g/kg.[248]

Much more attention has been directed toward the potential use of glutamine to boost the immune system of athletes than to provide energy to the muscles. As an important energy source for white blood cells, glutamine supplementation has been theorized to enhance immunity.[249] Some research suggests that athletes are more susceptible to infection than nonathletes, particularly during periods of overtraining. Overtraining has been associated with lower than normal plasma glutamine concentrations. While some research suggests that glutamine supplementation can improve markers of immune function and even decrease risk of infection, other studies have not produced similar results. More research is needed to provide a clearer picture of how training influences glutamine status and how glutamine supplementation affects immune function.

Glutathione is a tripeptide produced from glutamine, cysteine, and glycine. Glutathione is particularly important as part of an antioxidant defense system along with the selenium-dependent enzyme glutathione peroxidase and for the transport of neutral amino acids into cells via the gamma-glutamyl cycle. The importance of antioxidant defense systems for athletes is described in the entry for antioxidants.

Glutathione peroxidase converts the reduced form of glutathione to its oxidized form while reducing hydrogen peroxide and lipid peroxides. The elimination of these peroxides is important for preventing damage caused by these highly oxidative species.

Glycemic index (GI) is a measure of the effect that foods have on blood glucose. It is typically established by comparing the 2-hour blood glucose response of 50 g of carbohydrate from a test food to 50 g of carbohydrate from a standard food (either glucose or white bread). Glycemic index has potential implications in optimizing endurance performance. Burke et al. (1998) summarized the theories regarding the use of glycemic index for exercise.[250] These theories suggest that lower glycemic index foods may be of greatest value if consumed prior to exercise and that higher glycemic index foods may work best during exercise and for resynthesis of glycogen during recovery.

G

To date, few studies have actually assessed the role of glycemic index of foods consumed during exercise on physical performance. The basis that higher glycemic index foods are the best carbohydrate sources during exercise is currently founded primarily on theory. Many studies of a variety of types of carbohydrate sources, typically moderate or high in GI, have clearly demonstrated that carbohydrate consumption during exercise improves endurance performance.[251] In one study, feeding of a liquid vs. a solid meal resulted in differing effects of blood glucose and insulin at rest; however, during exercise these differences were not detected and the feedings affected exercise performance in a similar fashion.[252] With that in mind, since peak oxidation of carbohydrate typically occurs approximately 1 hour after feeding,[253] foods allowing for faster appearance of glucose in the blood are potentially of greatest benefit. However, many factors including individual variation in GI response and preference of food choice should not be discounted in the absence of strong evidence against feeding more moderate glycemic foods. Recent research comparing a high GI sports gel to raisins, which have a lower GI, suggested no difference in cycling performance.[254] Until more well-controlled comparisons of feedings of foods of various GI foods are available, recommendations regarding carbohydrate ingestion during exercise based on GI are unfounded.

The role of GI in preexercise feedings has been an area of much more comprehensive investigation. Although not all studies agree, likely due to differences in timing, quantity, and type of feeding including differences in GIs of test foods, and performance protocols, some research suggests that consumption of a lower GI food prior to exercise is more effective in enhancing performance than consumption of higher GI foods.[255–258] The improvement in performance has been suggested to be due to a reduction in hyperglycemia resulting in less hyperinsulinemia, as well as decreases in preexercise blood lactate concentration and maintenance of higher blood glucose and free fatty acid concentrations after commencing exercise. However, a number of studies have yielded no performance enhancement of lower vs. higher GI foods.[254,259–263] Of further interest, research by Burke et al. indicates that any potential effect of preexercise feedings of foods of various GIs is abolished when carbohydrate is also fed during exercise.[264]

Overall, GI may ultimately prove to be a useful tool for preevent feeding used to enhance endurance performance. Its usefulness to determine which carbohydrate sources to feed during exercise appears to be more questionable.

Glycerol (Figure G.5) is a water-soluble, 3-carbon alcohol molecule with hydroxyl groups attached to each carbon. It is an important intermediate in metabolism and can be used for the synthesis of carbohydrates as well as lipids. Perhaps most notably, glycerol is the 3-carbon backbone of mono-, di-, and triglycerides as well as glycero-

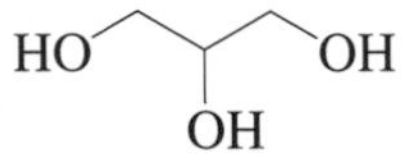

HO⌒⌒OH
OH

glycerol

FIGURE G.5

phosphatides, a group of phospholipids. Although glycerol can be eaten as part of many molecules, it is also synthesized within the body and is not an essential nutrient.

Since glycerol can be used for energy production as an intermediate molecule in glycolysis, its role as a fuel for exercise and potential ergogenic aid has been an area of interest. Most experts suggest that the conversion of glycerol to glucose is not sufficiently rapid and efficient to provide an ergogenic benefit during exercise; however, its supplementation has also been studied for its potential hydration capacity. As an extremely hydrophilic molecule, glycerol has been used to promote the retention of fluid within the body. Although not all studies agree,[265] several studies have supported the notion that consumption of exogenous glycerol can increase body water content, including producing increased plasma volume compared to plain water.[266,267] Maintenance of plasma volume and prevention of dehydration may improve athletic performance; however, fewer studies have actually demonstrated enhanced performance.

Glycerol-induced hyperhydration may also blunt the thermic response to exercise in the heat.[266] Some have also suggested that glycerol supplementation can prolong time to fatigue when exercise is performed at high ambient temperatures.[268,269]

The optimal dose and timing of glycerol supplementation has not been determined. Most studies have provided approximately 1 g of glycerol per kg body weight. Some research participants have reported adverse effects of glycerol supplementation, likely due to an osmotic effect. Symptoms reported include gastrointestinal distress such as nausea, bloating, and cramping, as well as headaches. Furthermore, if body weight gain is undesirable for competition, this could be considered an adverse side effect for some athletes.

Glycine (Figure G.6) is a nonessential amino acid synthesized from serine. Glycine, along with arginine and methionine, is used in the production of creatine, which has been demonstrated in many studies to enhance performance of repeated bouts of high intensity exercise. Due to its role in creatine production, glycine is sometimes touted as an ergogenic aid. To date no studies have supported an ergogenic effect of glycine. Early research by Hilsendager and Karpovich has suggested that glycine does not enhance short-term muscular endurance.[270]

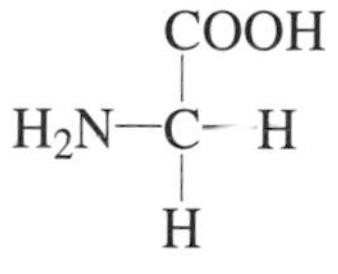

$$\begin{array}{c} COOH \\ | \\ H_2N-C-H \\ | \\ H \end{array}$$

glycine

FIGURE G.6

Glycogen (Figure G.7) is the storage form of carbohydrate in humans. It is a very compact, highly branched chain of glucose molecules linked together by α-1,4 and α-1,6 glycosidic bonds. The majority of glycogen stored in the body is located in the muscles and liver. In times of energy need, glycogen is broken down via glycogenolysis to produce glucose or glucose derivatives. Glycogen within a muscle cell must be used for energy within that cell, since glycogenolysis continues only until the production of the molecule glucose-6-phosphate, which cannot escape the cell, but can enter the glycolytic pathway for energy production. Glycogen within liver cells can be broken down to free glucose molecules, because the liver produces an enzyme

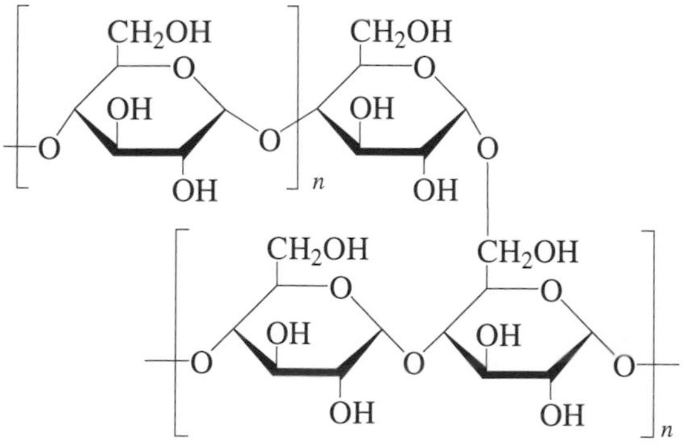

glycogen

FIGURE G.7

called glucose-6-phosphatase, which removes the phosphate molecule. Free glucose can leave the liver cell and travel via the circulation to tissues requiring production of energy.

Glycogen-sparing Many dietary techniques and supplements that have been used to improve endurance exercise performance are based on their potential glycogen-sparing properties. Adequate fuel substrates for exercise are critical for preventing fatigue. When liver glycogen is depleted during exercise, adequate production of glucose is not possible under conditions of intense physical activity; thus, hypoglycemia ensues and exhaustion occurs.

Consumption of exogenous carbohydrate before or during exercise has been a long-used technique that can spare glycogen and prevent fatigue from occurring earlier in exercise. Many other supplements and dietary strategies have been promoted as glycogen-sparing. Although evidence has supported the use of some of these, others have not been as successful. In some cases, glycogen-sparing has been demonstrated to occur but subsequent enhancements in performance were not detected. When that is the case, it is possible that the exercise protocol utilized failed to produce sufficient glycogen loss in control trials that could produce fatigue.

Glycolysis is the catabolism of glucose for energy. Glucose serves as a primary fuel for the body and is a highly preferred fuel for many cells including the central nervous system and red blood cells. When athletes need to rapidly produce energy from glucose during very strenuous exercise that can last for only a short time, a large proportion of that glucose will be metabolized anaerobically to produce ATP and the final product lactic acid. As the intensity of exercise decreases, aerobic glucose metabolism will predominate and although ATP will be produced less rapidly, the final product of glycolysis will be pyruvic acid, which can undergo further metabolism via the pyruvate dehydrogenase complex, followed by Krebs cycle and ultimately the electron transport system to produce additional ATP. Figure G.8 provides

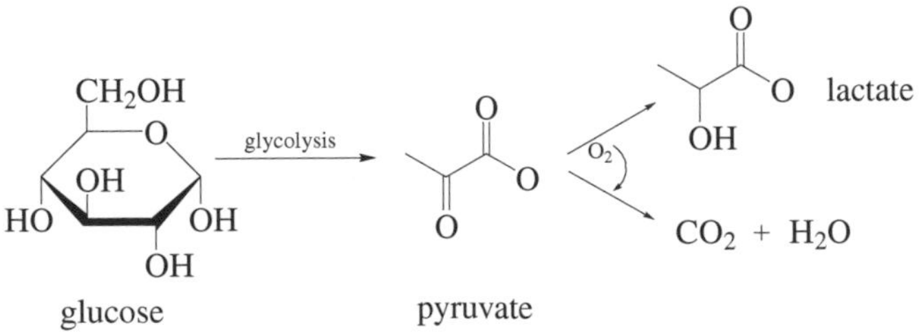

FIGURE G.8

a brief diagram of glycolysis, demonstrating that during anaerobic glycolysis, pyruvate is converted to lactate, but when oxygen is available, the pyruvate can be further catabolized.

GRAS *See* **Generally recognized as safe**

Green tea from the plant Camellia sinensis has become a popular herb due to its potential effects on chronic degenerative diseases (such as heart disease, cancer, etc.). The benefits of green tea have been ascribed to the antioxidative potential of it and its constituents (for example, tannins and catechins). To date, no studies have been published to evaluate green tea as an ergogenic aid in humans. Green tea preparations typically include caffeine, however, so the potential for enhanced performance with adequate consumption exists through this substance.

Growth hormone is a peptide hormone produced in the pituitary gland of the brain. It appears to exert its effects on growth by simulating the production of insulin-like growth factor-1 (IGF-1). Injections of human growth hormone are effective in stimulating weight gain in individuals who produced limited amounts of growth hormone endogenously, although some have suggested that the weight gain is due to water retention and the development of connective tissue. In exercisers who have normal levels of growth hormone, there is little evidence to suggest that increases in muscle synthesis and strength are likely to occur with administration of exogenous growth hormone. Furthermore, use of human growth hormone is banned by the International Olympic Committee.

Many nutrients and dietary supplements are marketed as anabolic substances due to their potential to elevate production of growth hormone. In most cases, evidence does not support a growth hormone stimulating effect from oral supplementation of these supplements. In other cases, growth hormone may be elevated under certain circumstances. In particular, when some amino acids are intravenously infused, growth hormone concentrations can be elevated. In a few studies, oral intake of some amino acids (such as arginine, lysine, and ornithine) has even produced elevations in growth hormone concentrations. Since actual injections of growth hormone are not likely to increase lean body mass and strength, however, it is unlikely that a dietary supplement marketed to elevate growth hormone will be of benefit for production of muscle tissue and strength in athletes.

Guarana (*Paulinia cupana*) is a plant containing significant amounts of chemical groups referred to as xanthines. Guarana typically contains theobromine (TB), theophylline (TP), and caffeine (CF) in most

G

preparations. These xanthines, particularly caffeine, are often attributed to the potential increased alertness from guarana supplementation.

Limited research is available regarding the potential interactive effects of guarana and exercise on metabolism. In one study 500 mg of a water extract of guarana per kg body weight was fed to mice.[271] Guarana increased blood glucose at rest and decreased liver glycogen content. It also suppressed exercise-induced hypoglycemia, but did not affect the blood glucose in epinephrine-induced mice. The authors concluded that guarana may promote liver glycogen breakdown, thereby preventing hypoglycemia. Although exercise performance was not assessed in these mice, such effects may translate to improved performance; however, since glycogen breakdown was higher, the converse may be true under some circumstances.

The are no human studies available regarding guarana as an ergogenic aid; however, with significant changes in caffeine status due to guarana use, the potential for improved performance exists via that mechanism. See the entry for caffeine for more information.

H

HDLs *See* **High density lipoproteins**

Heat injury can occur in athletes (as well as nonathletes) during exercise performed at high temperatures and high humidity. While heat injury can easily impair performance, more importantly, when ignored it can progress to the point of serious danger. Early indications of heat injury include dizziness, nausea, tingling sensations, and so forth, which can lead to heat stroke and even death if not kept in check. Physiological factors that often accompany heat injury include elevated body temperature, dehydration, and electrolyte imbalance. Many heat injuries can be prevented by adaptation to the thermal environment in which exercise will take place and consumption of adequate fluids prior to and during exercise. Additional precautions that can be taken to reduce the risk of heat injury include exercising during the coolest time of the day and wearing lightweight, comfortable clothing.

Hemoglobin is an iron-containing protein in red blood cells that transports oxygen from the lungs to tissues in exchange for carbon dioxide.

Herbs are typically defined simply as plants that do not have a woody stem. Herbal preparations are compounds produced from herbs that are thought to have medicinal or nutritional properties. Many herbs and their preparations are marketed as potential ergogenic aids as well as for other health properties. Most of these claims are unfounded, yet the sale of herbs remains big business.

Herbal preparations are regulated by the Dietary Supplement Health and Education Act enacted in 1994, which allows the sale of herbal preparations but does not allow the product label to include health claims. Several herb and herb-related entries are included in more detail throughout this book.

HGH *See* **Human growth hormone**

High density lipoproteins (HDLs) are lipid/protein complexes transported in the circulatory system. HDL particles are synthesized in the liver and to a lesser degree in the cells of the gastrointestinal tract. The primary role of HDL particles is the removal of cholesterol from lower density lipoproteins and tissues for transportation to the liver via the reverse cholesterol transport system.

The cholesterol in HDL particles is referred to as HDL-cholesterol (HDL-C). It is the fraction of cholesterol within HDL particles that is measured to determine a value for HDL-C. Since HDL particles are involved with reverse cholesterol transport, high levels of HDL-C are suggestive of low risk for heart disease.

Exercise training, and in some studies just single bouts of exercise, results in elevations in the serum concentrations of HDL-C.[133] Aerobic exercise appears to be more effective than anaerobic exercise in producing beneficial effects. Some scientists estimate that training that expends approximately 1000 kcals per week for at least 3 months is sufficient to provide elevations in HDL-C and thus protect against atherosclerosis.[133]

H

Histidine (Figure H.1) is an essential amino acid. In addition to serving as a building block for proteins, histidine is involved in biochemical reactions including histamine and carnosine production.

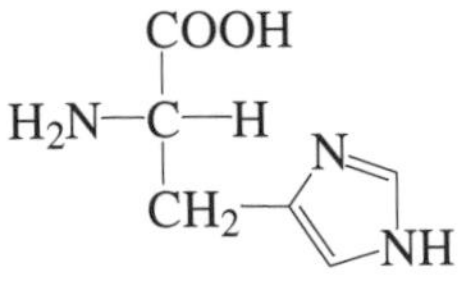

histidine

FIGURE H.1

HMB *See* **Beta-hydroxy-beta-methylbutyrate**

Hormone A hormone is a chemical produced in an endocrine gland that exhibits its effects at another site. Hormones can be polypeptides, amino acid derivatives, or lipid derivatives.

Hormone sensitive lipase (HSL) is an enzyme that mobilizes fatty acids from triglyceride stored in adipose cells in response to the actions of an array of hormones. Hormones known to activate HSL include epinephrine, norepinephrine, adrenocorticotropic hormone, thyroxine, thyroid-stimulating hormone, glucagon, and growth hormone.

Human growth hormone *See* **Growth hormone**

Hydration status refers to the regulation of water content and distribution within the body. The human body is approximately 60% water, which highlights its critical nature.[272] Water serves a host of life-supporting actions and if too much water is lost (dehydration), the body's well-being becomes compromised. Some principle roles for water in the body include: a) functioning as a medium for chemical reactions and transport of nutrients, metabolites, waste products, and other chemicals; b) cushioning and lubricating vital organs and tissues; c) synthesis of critical biomolecules; and d) thermoregulation. Therefore, dehydration can have detrimental effects on normal body functions.

The body loses water through a variety of mechanisms including urine production, fecal losses, perspiration, and "insensible" losses, which include water lost through the skin and respiration. Insensible losses are readily apparent to the individual. During physical activity the body loses a high percentage of its fluids via perspiration, which when evaporated from the skin serves to cool the body. Therefore, although fluid losses from sweat may compromise fluid status, it occurs in order to cool the body due to the increased heat production that occurs during exercise. In the process of perspiration, the body funnels a greater percentage of its blood flow to the capillaries of the skin, which contains sweat glands. Sweat is produced and secreted, which evaporates and cools the skin and the underlying blood, thereby reducing core body temperature. The rate of sweating depends on several factors including body size, exercise intensity, ambient temperature, humidity, and acclimation to the environment and exercise training.[273]

If fluid intake does not meet losses during exercise, a deficit occurs that could affect athletic performance. A water deficit increases plasma osmolality, which is sensed by the hypothalamus and stimulates thirst. Studies have suggested that the loss of less than 2% of body weight via dehydration can hinder athletic performance.[274] Therefore, preventing dehydration is a good way for athletes to maximize athletic performance and delay fatigue. Since some endurance athletes can lose between 1.5 to 1.8 liters or more during each hour of physical activity,[273] consuming plenty of fluid frequently during strenuous exercise must be a part of any training or competition regimen. Adequate hydration, especially during exercise performed in the heat, can assist in maintaining blood pressure and cardiac output, which are essential for adequate skin blood flow, sweat rates, and cooling.[275]

Dehydration can produce more serious consequences for the athlete and other individuals than merely a poor exercise performance.[275] At a fluid deficit of 5% of body water loss, some major symptoms of dehydration tend to occur. These include discomfort, lethargy, fatigue, loss of appetite, and nervousness. Dehydration levels of 7% or greater are extremely dangerous and might impair the ability to swallow. At 10% or more of fluid loss the ability to walk is impaired, and at over 20% the skin bleeds and cracks after which death is likely.

In humid environments the sweat does not evaporate as well as in drier conditions. Since much of the body's heat is lost through evaporative cooling, as heat production increases with exercise, body temperature increases, which further produces perspiration that once again does not allow for efficient cooling. If the ambient temperature is also high and exceeds body temperature, heat cannot be lost via radiation, which compounds the accumulation of body heat. Therefore, dehydration is more likely to occur under humid conditions, especially in the heat. Conditions of high temperature and high humidity might put the athlete at particularly high risk for heat injuries (such as heat cramps, heat exhaustion, heat stroke, etc.). Hyperthermia along with lower cardiac output produced during dehydration can hinder performance of high-intensity activities. The most severe form of heat injury, heat stroke, occurs when a failure of the temperature regulatory center in the hypothalamus occurs. The body core temperature can reach over 41°C.[275] Symptoms of heat stroke can include high temperature, headaches, nausea, dizziness, clumsiness, excessive inefficient sweating, and confusion, which can eventually progress to the loss of consciousness and when untreated even death.

Although less common, dehydration can also occur in cool environments. Fluid losses in the cold mainly occur via respiration; however, sweat losses can also contribute to dehydration if insulated cloths are being worn. In addition, low rates of fluids might be ingested due to a low thirst perception in a cold environment.[273]

Fluid requirements vary with several factors including sport/event, exercise intensity, duration of exercise bout, and climate; thus, it is impossible to provide all athletes with a single recommendation for fluid needed for competition. However, general recommendations of the American College of Sports Medicine, the American Dietetic Association, and Dietitians of Canada are to consume generous amounts of fluid in the 24 hours prior to the exercise.[273] In addition, the athlete should consume approximately 400 to 600 ml of fluid about 2 hours prior to exercise in order to optimize hydration while allowing any excess of fluids to be excreted before the exercise. In conditions of high ambient temperature, it is recommended to exceed these amounts and to consume approximately 400 to 600 ml again 20 minutes before the exercise to bring the body to a state of hyperhydration. Preexercise fluid uptake increases stomach volume, which is a major factor in optimizing gastric emptying.[210]

During competition or training the athlete should ingest between 150 to 350 ml of fluid every 15 to 20 minutes of exercise.[273] In order to maintain euhydration, the rate of fluid consumption should be equal to the rate of fluid loss. In prolonged events (lasting over 60 minutes) the athlete should consider ingesting fluids that contain carbohydrates at 4 to 8% concentration in order to supply an exogenous energy source. The guidelines also suggest that during prolonged exercise sodium should be added to the fluid at a rate of 0.5 to 0.7 g/L and to stimulate the thirst mechanism, thereby promoting adequate fluid intake and hydration. In particularly long events when fluid and body water replacement is high, sodium is also important for the prevention of hyponatremia. The entry for sports drinks provides additional information on this topic.

Athletes often fail to adequately maintain hydration during exercise in both long and short events. In this case a major role for the sports dietitian, athletic trainer, or related practitioner can be to optimize fluid intake by providing or suggesting the use of the most palatable fluids possible. Suggestions may include the use of 1) cool fluids (between 15 to 22°C); 2) flavored beverages; 3) sweetened beverages; and 4) beverages that include sodium. Studies have shown that each of these factors can enhance fluid intake, thus decreasing the likelihood of dehydration during an event.

Changes in body weight after exercise primarily indicate fluid losses and the adequacy of hydration during exercise. After exercise, the athlete should consume an amount of fluid that is equal to approximately 150% of body weight lost in order to meet fluid losses from sweat as well as subsequent urine production.[273] Well-hydrated individuals should produce relatively large amounts of urine that is light in color and free of a strong odor.[210] Ingesting sodium as part of fluid or food intake is commonly recommended after exercise in order to reduce diuresis and to help the rehydration process by maintaining plasma osmolality and thus thirst sensation.

Overall, adequate hydration during exercise is critical for optimal performance and to decrease risk of heat injury during training as well as competition. Athletes must be cognizant of their fluid losses and anticipate their fluid needs each time they exercise, particularly when in hot and humid conditions.

Hydroxymethylbutyrate *See* **Beta-hydroxy-beta-methylbutyrate**

Hyperglycemia is an elevation in the concentration of glucose in the blood above normal levels. Typically, when hyperglycemia occurs, insulin is released from the pancreas, which allows for the uptake of blood glucose by tissues such as muscle and adipose. When adequate insulin is not present or the body is not sensitive to its effects, hyperglycemia will likely not be transient. In some cases these conditions are referred to as type I and type II diabetes mellitus, respectively. For more information, see the entry for diabetes mellitus.

Hyperhydration The term hyperhydration is used to describe the process of consuming additional fluids to promote optimal hydration prior to an event. Recommendations for preevent fluid consumption are provided in the entry for hydration.

Hyperplasia *See* **Muscle hyperplasia**

Hypertension refers to abnormally high blood pressure. High blood pressure is related to an increased risk for heart disease and stroke. Obesity is a major contributor to hypertension; thus, exercise is particularly helpful for its prevention. Another mechanism by which exercise may prevent the development of or treat hypertension is hypothalamic-induced vasodilation. Hypertension can be caused by many factors and exercise is not always effective in preventing or treating all cases.

Hypertonic refers to greater than normal pressure. A hypertonic solution exerts more osmotic pressure than plasma. Hypertonic solutions ingested orally may promote the movement of water from the plasma to the gut, which can produce symptoms of gastrointestinal distress including nausea, cramping, and diarrhea.

Hypertrophy *See* **Muscle hypertrophy**

Hypervitaminosis *See* **Vitamin toxicity**

Hypoglycemia is a below normal concentration of glucose in the blood. Symptoms of hypoglycemia include dizziness, muscle weakness, fatigue, and hunger. When blood glucose concentration drops below normal, glucagon is secreted, which mobilizes glycogen from the liver to elevate blood glucose concentration.

In rare cases hypoglycemia can be a chronic condition. More often, hypoglycemia is a transient phenomenon. During exercise, particularly prolonged vigorous exercise, demands for carbohydrate for fuel can be high. While the liver and muscle can supply a relatively large amount of glycogen, during prolonged exercise those supplies can be depleted and gluconeogenesis (synthesis of glucose from noncarbohydrate sources) cannot occur at a rate sufficient to replenish the blood glucose. Ultimately, hypoglycemia and fatigue will occur. For this reason it is imperative for endurance athletes to consume a diet adequate in carbohdyrates to provide sufficient stores of glycogen. Likewise, it is important to consume adequate exogenous carbohydrates before and during exercise to prevent hypoglycemia.

In some athletes, consumption of a preexercise carbohydrate-rich meal (usually 15 to 60 minutes before exercise) can produce a sharp elevation in blood sugar. This increase results in production and release of insulin, which has a glucose-lowering effect. When exercise begins, the blood sugar concentration can be further decreased by increased tissue uptake of glucose. If the decrease is extreme, a transient hypoglycemia referred to as reactive hypoglycemia occurs. Since hypoglycemia can induce feelings of fatigue, exercise performance can be diminished in some athletes.[276]

Hypohydration is below adequate hydration status.

Hypokalemia is a below normal concentration of potassium in the blood.

Hyponatremia is a below normal concentration of sodium in the blood.

Hypotonic refers to a below normal pressure. A hypotonic solution will exert less osmotic pressure than that of plasma.

I

Immune system refers to the functional components of the body that help to fight off infections.

Incomplete protein An incomplete protein does not provide all of the essential amino acids in adequate proportions to meet demands for normal growth and development. Historically, plant proteins (except for soy proteins) and the animal protein gelatin have been classified as incomplete. See the entry for complete protein for more information.

Indispensable amino acid *See* **Essential amino acid**

Inosine is a nucleoside that in its monophosphate form (IMP) produces adenosine monophosphate (AMP), which can be further phosphorylated to eventually produce adenosine triphosphate (ATP). The connection between IMP and ATP synthesis has served as the basis for speculation that inosine supplementation can improve exercise performance, particularly for strength-related activities. It has also been suggested to improve endurance performance by shifting the oxygen dissociation curve to the left, allowing greater delivery of oxygen to the working muscle. Inosine is not an essential nutrient, since the body produces all the inosine it requires.

Research has not supported an ergogenic effect of inosine supplements.[277–279] Nor have studies provided evidence to suggest that metabolism is favorably altered in a way that under proper circumstances could improve performance. In fact, some studies have detected negative effects of inosine supplementation such as shorter time to fatigue during peak oxygen uptake cycling testing and poorer performance in intense, short-term activities.[278,279] Researchers speculate that inosine may impair performance by decreasing fast-twitch muscle function during high-intensity exercise.

Insulin is a peptide hormone synthesized in the beta cells of the pancreas. A primary function of insulin is the regulation of blood glucose, in which it most notably prevents blood glucose elevations by stimulating the uptake of glucose into the cell by glucose transporters. The primary transporter in skeletal muscle, the heart, and adipose cells is called the GLUT-4 transporter. When activated by insulin, GLUT-4 migrates to the cell membrane to allow the facilitated diffusion of glucose. Exercise also stimulates the function of GLUT-4 transporters;

thus, serum concentrations of insulin usually drop during exercise when food is not eaten.

In general, insulin is considered an anabolic hormone, because it directs metabolism toward biosynthetic reactions. For example, insulin stimulates glycogenesis (the formation of glycogen from glucose), protein synthesis from amino acids, and triglyceride production. While insulin is known for enhancing biosynthesis, it also increases activity of the phosphofructokinase, which is the enzyme involved in the rate-limiting step of glycolysis.

Intercellular water The water between cells is referred to as intercellular or interstitial fluid. Plasma, the fluid component of blood outside of the red blood cells, is a major percentage of the body's intercellular water. Intercellular water also includes water within the joints and pleura as well as fluids of the eyes and ears.

Interstitial fluid *See* **Intercellular water**

Intestinal absorption *See* **Absorption**

Intracellular water The water contained within the cells is referred to as intracellular water, which accounts for approximately 65% of the body's water.

Intravascular water The intercellular water within the blood vessels is considered the intravascular water. Adequate intravascular water is critical for health as well as efficient cardiac function during exercise.

Iodine is a micromineral that is mostly considered in conjunction with the thyroid gland and thyroid hormones. The principal source of iodine in the U.S. is iodized salt. Iodine is also found naturally in seafood as well as plants grown in iodine-rich soil. The main function of iodine is the production of thyroid hormones, which include iodine as part of their structures. Since iodine is needed for their production, deficiency can produce enlargement of the thyroid gland, referred to as goiter. The goiter is produced as a response to overstimulation of the thyroid gland by thyroid stimulating hormone. Iodine has not received attention as a potential ergogenic aid.

Ion An ion is a charged molecule. Ions with negative charges are called anions. Those with positive charges are called cations. Electrolytes in solutions are examples of ions.

Iron is a micromineral that is critical for the transport of oxygen within the body. This is accomplished within the circulation by the help of hemoglobin, which contains the heme molecule with a central iron atom. Transport of oxygen within the muscle occurs with the assistance of myoglobin, another heme-containing protein. Iron is also needed for the function of many enzymes including cytochromes, catalase, peroxidase, and others. In addition to functioning with cytochromes in the electron transport system, iron also shuttles electrons in the chain as part of iron-sulfur complexes.

Iron is found in foods in two primary forms: heme iron and nonheme iron. Heme iron is the more highly absorbed form with most estimates suggesting that about 25% of iron from heme can be absorbed. Meat, fish, and poultry contain heme iron as well as nonheme iron. Nonheme iron is absorbed at a much lower rate, although nonheme iron in the ferrous (reduced) form is more readily absorbed than ferric (oxidized) iron. Sources of nonheme iron other than meat, fish, and poultry include legumes, whole grain and enriched grain products, dark green vegetables, nuts, seeds, and others. To maximize absorption of iron from nonheme sources, individuals may consume meat, fish, or poultry, or foods rich in vitamin C along with the foods providing nonheme iron.

Iron deficiency has been classified into three different stages including iron storage deficiency, iron deficiency erythropoeisis, and iron deficiency anemia. Physical work capacity is diminished during iron deficiency anemia due to decreased ability of the body to transport and utilize oxygen; thus athletic performance can be hindered. The entry for iron deficiency anemia describes the deficiency of iron as well as its three stages in more detail. See the entry for sports anemia for information regarding the potential influence of physical activity on the development or apparent development of anemia.

Iron deficiency anemia Anemia is a term used to describe a number of conditions in which red blood cell concentration or function is below normal. Iron deficiency anemia is caused by low dietary intake of iron and is characterized by small, lightly colored red blood cells with low concentrations of hemoglobin. Physical work capacity is diminished during iron deficiency anemia due to decreased ability of the body to transport and utilize oxygen.

In general, iron deficiency can exist in three stages. Iron deficiency anemia is the most severe form and occurs in the third stage. A person with stage 1 iron deficiency is predisposed to true anemia but does not exhibit its physical or biochemical signs except for a low concentration of ferritin in the serum, as well as in the bone marrow, spleen, and liver, where iron is stored as ferritin. This stage is referred to as iron storage deficiency and can progress to iron deficiency erythropoeisis (stage 2). Although physical work capacity and red blood cells remain normal in stage 2, the body responds to the lack of iron in the diet by producing protoporphyrin, the precursor to heme, which does not contain iron. Synthesis of the molecule that transports iron in the circulation (transferrin) also increases, which increases the total iron binding capacity in the blood and decreases transferring saturation.

Adequate intake of iron is necessary to prevent iron deficiency anemia and its predisposition. Since normally menstruating women of childbearing age have the highest dietary requirement for iron due to monthly blood loss, they are particularly susceptible to iron deficiency; thus, in athletics, women are more susceptible to iron deficiency than men. While these women are most susceptible, all athletes must ensure adequate dietary iron for optimal performance. Foods richest in iron and providing the mostly highly available form (heme iron) include meat, fish, and poultry. Some iron in the nonheme form is also available in these foods as well as many others. These foods include legumes, whole grain and enriched grain products, dark green vegetables, nuts, seeds, and others. Although these foods provide less iron that is not absorbed as well, absorption efficiency can be increased when the foods are consumed with foods rich in vitamin C or with meat, fish, and poultry.

Isokinetic In exercise, the term isokinetic is used to refer to resistance-training exercises that are performed at the same speed throughout the muscular contraction. Many studies assessing the effects of dietary interventions on strength utilize special machines that allow this type of movement.

Isoleucine (Figure I.1) is a branched-chain, essential amino acid. It is needed for synthesis of proteins and can be used for energy production within the muscle cell as well. Metabolism of isoleucine in the muscle results in the production of acetyl CoA and propionyl CoA. The acetyl CoA can be further metabolized for energy production via Krebs cycle. Additionally, within just a few biochemical steps, the propionyl CoA can be converted to succinyl CoA, which is an intermediate of Krebs cycle.

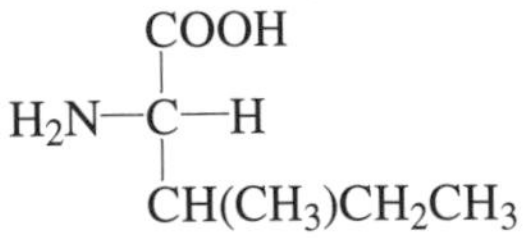

$$COOH$$
$$H_2N-C-H$$
$$CH(CH_3)CH_2CH_3$$

isoleucine

FIGURE I.1

Since catabolism of branched-chain amino acids may be important in producing central fatigue, as described in a separate entry, many studies have examined their ergogenic potential. While some researchers have provided individual branched-chain amino acids to their participants, most have fed the compounds as mixtures. Research on the potential ergogenic benefits of their supplementation is described in the entry for branched-chain amino acids.

Isometric In exercise, the term isometric is used to refer to resistance-training exercises in which the muscle is static (neither shortens nor lengthens) throughout the contraction. A common example of this type of exercise is the wall sit, in which a person stands against a wall with the knees and hips at opposite 45° angles.

Isotonic refers to "the same pressure." In nutrition, isotonic beverages exert the same osmotic pressure as plasma. In exercise, the term isotonic is used to refer to resistance-training exercises in which the same pressure is applied throughout the muscular contraction, although in truth, as biomechanics change throughout the range of contraction, the resistance encountered can vary throughout the exercise. Isotonic exercises can be divided into those that produce either concentric or eccentric contractions, which are described in separate entries.

I

J

Joule A joule is a unit for measuring energy. The term joule is used in preference to calorie in many countries. One calorie is the equivalent of 4.184 joules.

K

Kelp There is no research available regarding the use of kelp as an ergogenic aid. Although several varieties of kelp have been analyzed for their nutritional contents, there is no reason to believe that kelp possesses any properties different from those of the nutrients it possesses. Kelp is generally considered rich in iodine and vitamins. Iodine supplementation is not known to affect exercise performance. Separate entries for each vitamin describe their potential uses as supplements for athletic performance. Although kelp is somewhat commonly used as a vitamin and mineral supplement, some concerns regarding its safety due to contaminants have been raised.[280]

Ketones are organic compounds containing keto-groups, which in general are characterized by an oxygen molecule double bonded to carbon. In metabolism, ketones and ketoacids are produced from acetyl CoA. Acetone is a ketone and acetoacetate and beta-hydroxybutyrate are ketoacids produced in metabolism. Ketones can be utilized for energy by red blood cells and tissues of the central nervous system at times when glucose is unavailable. When ketone production increases to a rate greater than the rate of catabolism, a state of ketosis can occur, which is described in that entry.

Ketosis occurs when the rate of ketone production is greater than the rate of ketone catabolism. Ketone synthesis can be increased by many factors including starvation, a low carbohydrate diet, uncontrolled diabetes mellitus, and ingestion of large amounts of medium-chain triglycerides (MCT). In each of the first three, carbohydrate is unavailable for the production of pyruvate, which can produce oxaloacetate. Oxaloacetate is the 4-carbon molecule that accepts the two acetate carbons of acetyl CoA to begin Krebs cycle. Decreased production of oxaloacetate leads to acetyl CoA accumulation, which results in the production of acetoacetyl CoA from the joining of two acetyl CoA molecules. Acetoacetyl CoA produces the ketoacid acetoacetate, which produces acetone (a ketone) and beta-hydroxybutyrate (another ketoacid). MCT ingestion can also promote ketosis, especially when fed as part of a low carbohydrate diet, since medium-chain fatty acids are primarily converted to ketones upon delivery to the liver following absorption.

Although ketosis can progress to a dangerous level, it occurs in the lack of available carbohydrate as a way to provide the red blood cells and tissues of the central nervous system with an alternate fuel source in the absence of adequate glucose. Ketones can accumulate at higher than normal levels under many circumstances, but typically are only considered harmful when produced to an extent that acid–base balance becomes disturbed. When pH drops to a dangerously low level, metabolic derangements occur that can result in dehydration, loss of blood volume, and eventually coma and death.

During exercise ketone production and utilization is increased, providing athletes with an additional source of energy. While little research is available to determine the impact of ketosis on athletic performance, many have speculated that it could be impaired due to a lack of available glucose for energy. However, research has suggested that a diet extremely low in carbohydrate and high in fat that produced a state of ketosis did not impair exercise performance.[281]

Kilocalorie A kilocalorie (kcal), also written as a Calorie, is equal to 1000 calories and is the primary term used in the U.S. to describe the measurement of energy within a food or expended by the body. Since one calorie is typically defined as the amount of heat required to raise 1 g of water by 1°C, one kilocalorie is the heat required to raise 1 kg of water 1°C. The term used most commonly internationally to describe energy is the joule (j). One Calorie (kcal) is the equivalent of 4.184 Joules (kj). When describing daily food intake or energy expenditure, the term megajoule (Mj) is often used.

Krebs cycle (also known as the citric acid cycle or the tricarboxylic acid [TCA] cycle) is a metabolic pathway that is instrumental in obtaining energy from macronutrients. In this cyclic pathway (Figure K.1), oxaloacetate, produced from pyruvate, accepts the 2 carbons of acetate from acetyl CoA (produced primarily from carbohydrates and fats via glycolysis and beta-oxidation, respectively) producing the 6-carbon molecule citrate. Following several steps, citrate is ultimately converted back to the 4-carbon molecule oxaloacetate with the loss of 2 carbons as carbon dioxide. The oxaloacetate is now available to accept

2 more carbons from acetyl CoA and continue the cycle. Also produced in Krebs cycle is guanosine triphosphate (GTP) and the energy-producing equivalents NADH + H+ and FADH$_2$. Like adenosine triphoshate (ATP), GTP possesses a high-energy bond that when cleaved can produce free energy similarly to that of ATP. NADH + H+ and FADH$_2$ are further metabolized via the electron transport system to produce ATP.

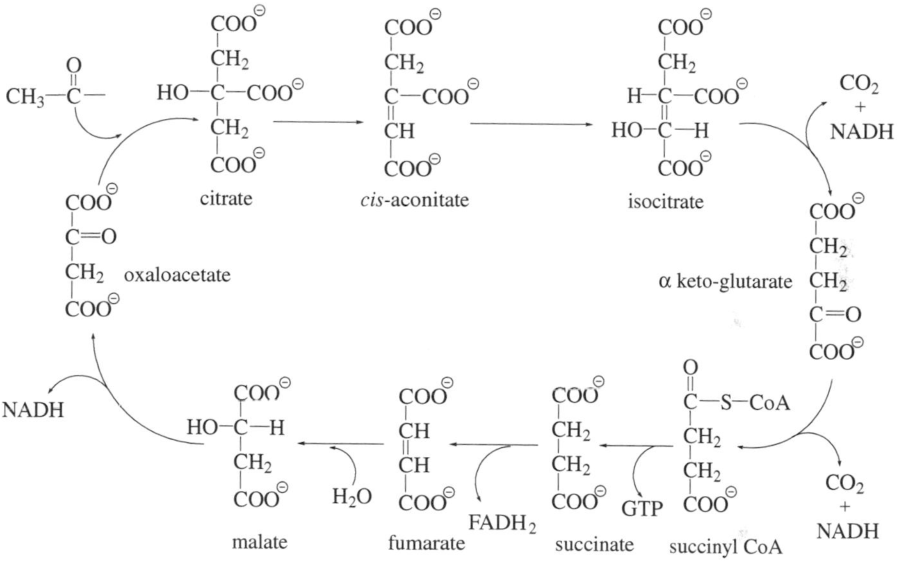

FIGURE K.1

L

Lactate *See* **Lactic acid**

Lactic acid (Figure L.1), also referred to as lactate, is the final product formed in anaerobic glycolysis. It is produced by the addition of hydrogen molecules to pyruvate. During recovery from exercise, the enzyme lactic acid dehydrogenase converts lactate back to pyruvate, producing NADH+ H+. The pyruvate produced can be used to produce glucose via gluconeogenesis.

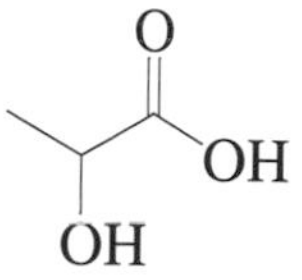

lactic acid

FIGURE L.1

Lactate has also been used as a potential ergogenic aid. Some have theorized that chronic ingestion of lactate could produce an adaptation that would enhance the body's ability to buffer lactate accumulation during exercise, thereby enhancing performance during strenuous exercise. However, research has not supported this theory.[282] Lactate as part of a sports beverage has also failed to enhance performance in comparison to carbohydrate when fed alone or in combination with carbohydrate.[283]

Polylactate, lactic acid combined with an amino acid, has also been studied for its ergogenic potential. Manufacturers have claimed that polylactate can enhance endurance. Research, however, has been equivocal regarding its usefulness. One study suggested that when 0.75 g/100 ml of polylactate was added to a 6.25% glucose polymer solution, feedings at the rate of 3 g carbohydrate per kg of body weight every 20 minutes until fatigue, failed to enhance performance compared to a 7% glucose polymer solution containing no polylactate.[284] In another study, a 7% solution containing an 80:20 mixture of polylactate and lactate produced an enhancement in the blood buffering capacity, but not differences in ratings of perceived exertion.[285] However, no data on exercise performance were reported.

Lactoovovegetarian A lactoovovegetarian will consume dairy foods and eggs in addition to plant foods, but will not consume meat, fish, or poultry.

Lactose (Figure L.2) is a disaccharide produced from the monosaccharides glucose and galactose. It is the primary sugar found in milk. Lactose is digested to its complementary monosaccharides by the enzyme lactase, which is secreted at the brush border of the small intestine. If inadequate amounts of lactase are produced by the body, lactose intolerance occurs, in

CH₂OH

OH   α-form

lactose

FIGURE L.2

which the individual cannot tolerate large (or sometimes even small) amounts of lactose. See the entry for lactose intolerance for more information.

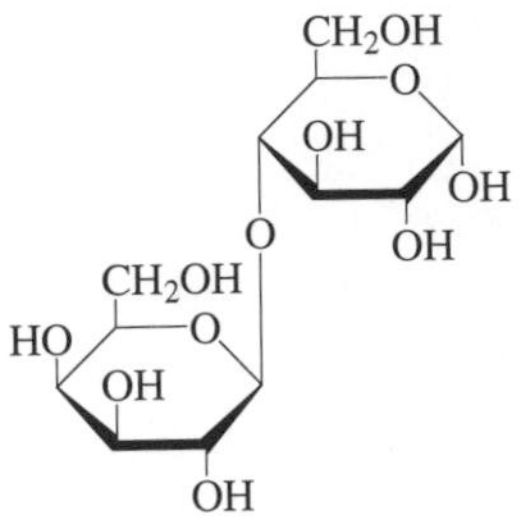

Lactose intolerance occurs when there is insufficient production of the enzyme lactase to digest the simple sugar lactose. When lactose goes partially or largely unabsorbed, several adverse reactions occur. One effect of lactose intolerance is diarrhea. Since lactose is a hydrophilic molecule, if unabsorbed it can pull water into the gastrointestinal tract producing an osmotic diarrhea. Furthermore, the unabsorbed lactose can be fermented by bacteria in the colon, which produces gas. Together, these effects also produce symptoms of bloating, cramping, and abdominal pain. Athletes with lactose intolerance must be careful not to consume milk-based beverages during competition.

Lactovegetarian A lactovegetarian will consume dairy foods in addition to plant foods, but will not consume meat, fish, poultry, or eggs.

LDLs *See* **Low density lipoproteins**

Lean body mass (often referred to as fat-free mass) is the portion of the body that is not associated with the adipose tissue. The muscles, bones, and visceral organs account for the majority of the body's lean mass.

Lecithin also known as phosphatidyl choline, is an important emulsifier in foods and within the body. Lecithin is critical for the formation of cell membranes. It also participates in important chemical reactions in the body, perhaps most notably along with the enzyme lecithin:cholesterol acyl transferase (LCAT), which is involved in the reverse cholesterol transport system.

Dietary lecithin also provides choline to the body. Choline and lecithin have been marketed for their ergogenic potential, primarily due to choline's association with acetylcholine and muscular contraction. While choline deficiency in those unable to produce adequate amounts of choline will almost certainly prevent optimal athletic performance, no studies have established a true ergogenic effect of choline or lecithin.

Legume A legume is a plant that has nodules on its roots containing nitrogen-fixing bacteria. Peas and beans that are typically dried prior to preparation are examples of legumes in the diet.

Leptin is a protein hormone synthesized from the *ob* gene in the adipose tissue and taken up by the brain where it inhibits the action of neuropeptide Y (NPY). Leptin appears to be important for normal reproductive function as well as for controlling body weight through regulation of appetite and energy expenditure. Leptin deficiency produces increased food intake and decreased energy expenditure resulting in obesity. Interestingly, obese individuals often have elevated concentrations of leptin, suggesting that leptin sensitivity and function are reduced. In animal models,[286] and more recently humans,[287] exogenous leptin administration has produced marked weight loss.

Leucine (Figure L.3) is a branched-chain, essential amino acid. It is needed for synthesis of proteins and can be used for energy production within the muscle cell as well. Metabolism of leucine in the muscle results in the production of acetyl CoA and acetoacetic acid. The acetyl CoA can be further metabolized for energy production via Krebs cycle.

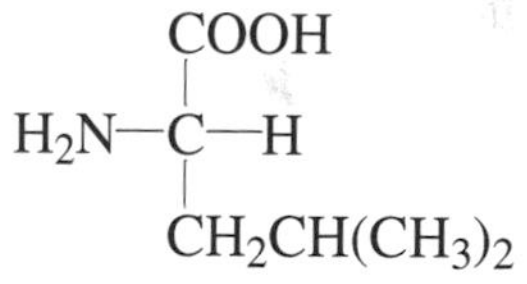

$$COOH$$
$$H_2N-C-H$$
$$CH_2CH(CH_3)_2$$

leucine

FIGURE L.3

Additionally, within just a few biochemical steps, the acetoacetic acid can also be converted to acetyle CoA for addtional metabolism through Krebs cycle.

Since catabolism of branched-chain amino acids may be important in producing central fatigue, as described in a separate entry, many studies have examined their ergogenic potential. While some researchers have provided individual branched-chain amino acids to their participants, most have fed the compounds as mixtures. Research on the potential ergogenic benefits of their supplementation is described in the entry for branched-chain amino acids.

Leucine also appears to be particularly important for protein synthesis in exercisers. These roles were recently reviewed by Layman.[288] His review indicates that leucine is responsible for much of the protein synthesis that occurs with protein or amino acid supplementation following exercise. Leucine apparently accomplishes this as a) a substrate for protein synthesis; b) a fuel for metabolism; and c) a metabolic, intracellular signal that amplifies insulin function. Research regarding postexercise protein and amino acid supplementation in maximizing protein synthesis is described in the protein entry.

Levulose *See* **Fructose**

Limiting amino acid A limiting amino acid is an essential amino acid in a dietary protein that provides the lowest amount in proportion to the amino acid contents of an equal amount of egg protein.

Linoleic acid is an essential fatty acid with 18 carbons and 2 double bonds. Richest dietary sources include a variety of vegetable oils such as soybean, corn, safflower, cottonseed, sunflower seed, and peanut oil. When not present in adequate amounts in the diet, linoleic acid deficiency can produce dermatitis, decreased growth or weight loss, organ dysfunction, and abnormal reproductive status. See entries for essential fatty acids and omega-6 fatty acids for more information.

Linolenic acid is available as two different structures, both with 18 carbons and 3 double bonds. Alpha-linolenic acid is an omega-3 fatty acid that is essential in the diet; whereas gamma-linolenic acid is an omega-6 fatty acid that can be synthesized from linoleic acid by the addition of a double bond by the delta-9-desaturase enzyme. Richest dietary sources of alpha-linolenic acid include a variety of vegetable oils such as soybean, flaxseed, linseed, and walnut oils. Alpha-linolenic acid deficiency can produce dermatitis, decreased growth or weight loss, organ dysfunction, and abnormal reproductive status. See entries for essential fatty acids and omega-6 fatty acids for more information.

Lipids *See* **Fats**

Lipoproteins are compound lipids deriving their name from their two primary components: lipids and proteins. The proteins that are constituents of lipoproteins are called apolipoproteins, sometimes shortened as apoproteins. Apoproteins serve a variety of roles including allowing transport of lipids within an aqueous environment, receptor recognition, and participating in a variety of biochemical reactions. Many lipids are transported as parts of the various lipoproteins. The lipids producing the majority of mass in a lipoprotein include triglycerides, cholesterol, cholesterol esters, and phospholipids. Primary classes of lipoproteins include chylomicrons, very low density lipoproteins (VLDL), low density lipoproteins (LDL), and high density lipoproteins (HDL).

Chylomicrons are triglyceride-rich lipoproteins produced in the cells of the gastrointestinal tract from the lipids consumed in the diet. They are absorbed via the lymphatic system and transported to the subclavian vein, which empties in the vena cava, allowing for distribution throughout the circulatory system by the heart. After a meal, much of the triglycerides in the chylomicrons are removed by the action of lipoprotein lipase, which hydrolyzes the triglyceride thus producing fatty acids, monoglycerides, and diglycerides, which are taken up by peripheral tissues. This process yields a chylomicron remnant with a lower concentration of triglyceride, which can be taken up by the liver.

VLDL, LDL, and HDL are produced primarily in the liver, although some HDL particles are produced in the cells of the gastrointestinal tract. Once synthesized, VLDL particles (which are also triglyceride-rich) are secreted into the circulation from the liver. They are metabolized in a manner similar to chylomicrons, ultimately producing LDL particles. LDL, which is less rich in triglyceride and contains high concentrations of cholesterol, is responsible for the majority of cholesterol transport. Since LDL particles are cholesterol-rich and can be deposited within the intima of the blood vessels, they are considered atherogenic at high concentrations, especially when oxidized. The primary role of HDL particles is to remove cholesterol from lower-density lipoproteins and ultimately deliver the lipids back to the liver through the process of the reverse cholesterol transport.

Separate entries are provided regarding total cholesterol in all lipoproteins in serum as well as high-density lipoproteins and low-density lipoproteins. The benefits of exercise for each of these lipids are described as well.

Liquid meals Many athletes consume liquid meals, also known as meal replacement beverages, because they are convenient and can often be consumed closer to the time of the event or training session. For example, many endurance sports, such as running, cycling, and triathlon, have early start times, which prevent athletes from consuming solid meals prior to competition, since these foods can potentially delay digestion and absorption relative to some liquid meals. Another advantage is that many available formulas produce little residue in the gastrointestinal tract. Most meal replacement beverages are available in cans, which is extremely convenient and eliminates the need for preparation.

Liquid meals consumed prior to competition or training should meet certain criteria. For example, a liquid meal should be rich in carbohydrates, but low in fat and fiber. Recent research also suggests that moderate amounts of protein may be useful and produces few if any adverse effects.[103] Liquid meals designed as supplements for specific medical conditions that are particularly high in fat, fiber, or protein should be avoided. Some commercial formulas are specifically designed with athletes in mind and, if so, are usually formulated to meet the necessary characteristics. Some athletes may prefer to prepare their own formula, such as a "smoothie," from scratch, which can be a cost-effective, nutrient-rich alternative. Since these meals can be made from natural, wholesome foods, if prepared properly they may actually be a preferred alternative to more highly processed canned beverages and could be included as a healthier alternative for daily training.

Liquid meals can also be used after exercise for quick replenishment of lost energy stores and to provide protein for muscle synthesis. A liquid meal is not likely to offer a metabolic advantage over solid food, but may be a convenient alternative. Athletes who have difficulty eating solid foods after exercise may prefer a liquid meal to prevent gastrointestinal distress.

Liver glycogen *See* **Glycogen**

Long-chain fatty acids Fatty acids with chain lengths of 12 or more carbons are usually considered long-chain fatty acids. However, some references classify lauric acid, which has 12 carbons, as a medium-chain fatty acid.

Low density lipoproteins (LDLs) are within a group of complexes of lipids and proteins that are particularly rich in cholesterol. Their primary function is cholesterol transport. LDL particles are produced in the catabolism of VLDL by the action of lipoprotein lipase. VLDL are transiently converted to intermediate density lipoproteins (IDL) during this process.

The cholesterol in LDL particles is referred to as LDL-cholesterol (LDL-C). It is the fraction of cholesterol within LDL particles that is measured to determine a value for LDL-C. Since LDL can be deposited in the intima of arteries, high concentrations of LDL-C in the serum are associated with increased risk for heart disease. When LDLs are oxidized, they are particularly atherogenic.

Exercise training, and in some studies just single bouts of exercise, produces decreases in the serum concentrations of LDL-C.[133] Aerobic exercise appears to be more effective than anaerobic exercise in producing beneficial effects.

Lysine (Figure L.4) is an essential amino acid that is integral for protein formation. Along with vitamin C, lysine is particularly important for the formation of collagen. Lysine has been marketed for its potential augmentation of growth hormone, thereby enhancing production of muscle. As reviewed by Williams, most available research does not support a role for lysine supplementation in raising growth hormone

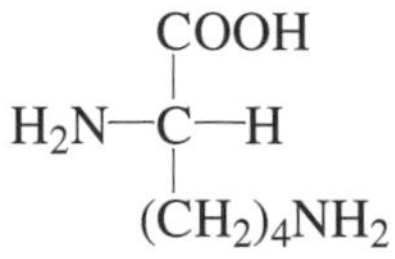

$$COOH$$
$$|$$
$$H_2N-C-H$$
$$|$$
$$(CH_2)_4NH_2$$

lysine

FIGURE L.4

concentration.[289] As described in the entry for growth hormone, even direct injections of growth hormone are unlikely to enhance muscle synthesis in those who produce adequate levels endogenously.

L

M

Macromineral A macromineral can be defined as a mineral that is required in amounts greater than or equal to 100 mg per day or a mineral that constitutes 0.01% or more of the weight of the body.

Macronutrient The term macronutrient has been defined in a variety of ways. Some refer to macronutrients as any nutrient required in large amounts. Others limit the term to nutrients required in large amounts that also provide energy in the diet. These constituents include fats, proteins, carbohydrates, and alcohol. In some cases alcohol is excluded when discussing macronutrients. If the ability to provide energy from the diet is not included as part of the classification, water is also considered a macronutrient and some may include fiber.

Magnesium is a macromineral that is essential to normal health. Common dietary sources of magnesium include legumes, whole grain cereals, green leafy vegetables, and nuts. Much of the magnesium in the body is located in the bones, where it provides structure and rigidity to the bone and also acts as a reservoir for nonbone-related functions. These functions are varied and primarily related to roles as a cofactor for many enzymes. Some of the many biochemical needs for magnesium include nucleic acid and protein synthesis, creatine phosphate formation, glycolysis, Krebs cycle, and the regulation of normal blood pressure. Deficiency of magnesium can produce symptoms such as nausea, vomiting, muscle weakness, and spasms. It may also be related to the development of chronic diseases including hypertension, diabetes mellitus, and cardiovascular disease.

In athletes, magnesium supplementation has been theorized to have a range of effects from increasing maximal oxygen consumption to improving muscular strength and lean body mass. As reviewed by Williams,[290] the potential benefits of magnesium supplementation in adequately nourished athletes appear to be minimal; however, a few studies have provided some evidence that is worthy of follow-up research. In an interesting case study of a tennis player, magnesium supplementation apparently relieved muscular cramping.[291] Research is needed to sort out whether the improvements detected by some research are simply the result of magnesium replenishment in deficient athletes or if magnesium requirements for optimal performance are higher than typical dietary recommendations.

Ma huang is an herb also known as *Ephedra sinica* that is common to Chinese medicine. The component of ma huang that has received the most attention with relation to athletic performance is ephedrine. See the entry on ephedrine for more information on its potential use as an ergogenic aid.

Malabsorption occurs when any nutrient is not absorbed normally. This can occur when digestion is inadequate to allow for absorption, as with the lack of an adequate digetive enzyme, or when the cells of the gastrointestinal tract are unable to properly absorb nutrients.

Malnutrition occurs when one or more nutrients is deficient in the diet or eaten in excess. In the case of deficiency, an essential nutrient or total energy may be deficient in the diet. In the case of excess, many nutrients can produce toxic effects and excess energy intake can cause obesity. The effects of micronutrient deficiency or toxicity are specific to each nutrient.

Maltodextrins are polymers of glucose molecules linked by glycosidic bonds. Maltodextrins, some times referred to as glucose polymers, are produced by partial hydrolysis of starch molecules, which are longer polymers of glucose. Maltodextrins have theoretical advantages over simpler carbohydrates due to the larger size of particles in maltodextrins, which decreases the osmotic load of a solution compared to a solution containing an equal amount of energy from simpler sugars. As reviewed by Lamb and Brodowicz, research has determined that this property may increase the rate of gastric emptying and allow for faster glucose and water absorption in the intestinal tract.[292] Available evidence, however, typically suggests that maltodextrins offer no advantage over other carbohydrates for exercise performance.

Maltose (Figure M.1) is a disaccharide produced from two units of glucose linked by alpha-1,4 glycosidic bonds. It is found in malted milk products as well as sweet potatoes and pears, and in lower amounts in other fruits, vegetables, and grain products, as well as honey. Maltose is primarily digested to its complementary monosaccharides primarily by the enzyme maltase, which is secreted at the brush border of the small intestine.

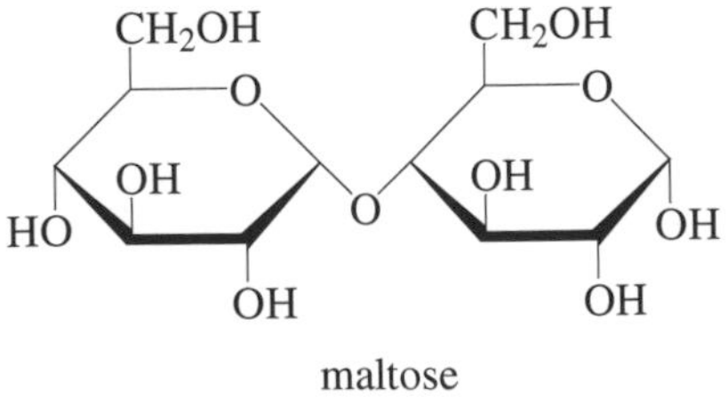

maltose

FIGURE M.1

Manganese is an essential micromineral that has been less well studied than many others. Dietary sources include legumes, whole grains, some fruits, and meat, fish, and poultry. Manganese has been linked to brain function and is important for normal function of several enzymes, including a manganese-dependent superoxide dismutase, which provides an antioxidant defense. It is also required for the production of urea. Although manganese has some role in the antioxidant defense of the body, its potential use in athletes has not been assessed.

Maximal aerobic capacity *See* **Maximal oxygen consumption**

Maximal oxygen consumption (VO_{2max}) is sometimes referred to as maximal aerobic capacity. It is determined by assessing the body's ability to maximally utilize oxygen during a graded exercise test. Intensity of physical activity is often expressed as a percentage of VO_{2max}.

MCT oil *See* **Medium-chain triglycerides**

Medium-chain fatty acids Fatty acids with chain lengths of between 6 to 10 carbons are considered medium-chain fatty acids. Additionally, some references classify lauric acid, which has 12 carbons, as a medium-chain fatty acid as well.

Medium-chain triglycerides (**MCTs**) MCT oil, currently marketed as an ergogenic aid, is theorized to enhance endurance performance because their medium-chain fatty acids are readily absorbed[293] and quickly metabolized independent of long-chain fatty acid transport mechanisms.[294] While long-chain fatty acids are absorbed into the cells of the gut, reesterified to glycerol, and packaged as part of chylomicrons for absorption via the lymphatic system, medium-chain fatty acids tend to be absorbed directly into the portal circulation for transport to the liver. In the liver, they are primarily converted to ketones and used for energy or secreted to the general circulation for uptake by peripheral tissues.[295] Researchers have suggested that the ketones produced can provide an alternate fuel source that could preserve muscle and liver glycogen during exercise.

Several studies have assessed the effects of acute feeding of MCT before and during exercise on endurance performance. Significant glycogen sparing has not been observed in these acute feeding studies; however, Van Zyl et al. did observe a significant improvement in cycling endurance with acute feeding of carbohydrate plus MCT oil vs. carbohydrate or MCT oil alone.[296] The results of this study have been criticized, however, since the energy content of the combination feeding was greater than that in the trials of the separate components. Regardless, MCT oil may offer a potential source of energy to the athlete, which can be included in addition to carbohydrates. Overall, most studies assessing the potential ergogenic effects of acute MCT

M

oil feedings vs. isocaloric carbohydrate feedings have provided no evidence of endurance enhancement.[297,298] In fact, Jeukendrup et al. observed that intake of MCT (85 g) during exercise negatively affected performance, and that the negative effect was associated with complaints of gastrointestinal distress.[299]

Fushiki and associates observed that chronic ingestion (2 to 6 weeks) of MCT (17% total dietary kcal) by both trained and untrained mice caused glycogen sparing and produced significantly greater swimming endurance capacity.[300] The authors suggested that adaptation to MCT oil feeding can upregulate enzymes of lipid metabolism, which may play a part in glycogen sparing.

Since long-term adaptation to MCT oil has been demonstrated to enhance lipid metabolism in animals, Misell et al. conducted similar research in humans.[301] Overall, they demonstrated that trained runners fed MCT oil for 2 weeks exhibited little differences in physiology and endurance performance compared to when supplementing the diet with corn oil after fasting. Although these data do not corroborate the results displayed in animals, it is unclear whether the mice in the study by Fushiki et al. were tested for endurance in a fasted or fed condition.[300] Future human research should examine the effects of a combination of long-term plus acute MCT oil ingestion on performance.

Megadose In general, a megadose is a high intake of a vitamin or mineral. Some experts have defined a megadose as at least 10 times the recommended quantity. Others have suggested that a medadose exceeds the Tolerable Upper Intake Level (UL) established by the Food and Nutrition Board of the National Academy of Sciences.

Metabolic rate The metabolic rate is the rate of energy expenditure. Basal metabolic rate refers to energy expenditure at rest, just after waking.

Metabolism refers to the biochemical reactions and processes producing catabolism and anabolism within the body.

Methionine (Figure M.2) is an essential amino acid containing sulfur that is needed for production of proteins. Methionine serves as a methyl group donor in many reactions and is needed for the synthesis of the nonessential amino acid cysteine. A related chemical, S-adenosyl methionine, has become a popular dietary supplement in the past few years and is described briefly in a separate entry.

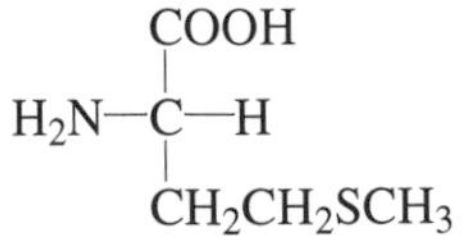

$$
\begin{array}{c}
COOH \\
| \\
H_2N-C-H \\
| \\
CH_2CH_2SCH_3
\end{array}
$$

methionine

FIGURE M.2

Micromineral A micromineral can be defined as a mineral that is required in amounts less than 100 mg per day or a mineral that constitutes less than 0.01% of the weight of the body.

Micronutrient The term micronutrient refers to nutrients required in minute amounts. It is used to describe vitamins and minerals as a group of nutrients.

Minerals From a nutritional perspective, minerals are inorganic elements that are required for normal growth and metabolism. Minerals required in large amounts are referred to as macrominerals, while those required in only small amounts are considered microminerals. Some experts refer to microminerals as trace or ultratrace minerals or elements depending upon their level of requirement. The functions of minerals vary, but typically include forming an important part of a chemical structure or participating as a cofactor for biochemical reactions.

Although many minerals have been marketed as ergogenic aids, well-designed studies have largely failed to support the need for supplementation of any mineral in nondeficient athletes. For all essential minerals, it is very likely that a clinical deficiency will impair athletic performance.

It is possible that under certain circumstances and with the correct dosage and timing of intake that some minerals could some day prove to be ergogenic. However, with today's state of science, with the possible exception of the need for electrolyte replacement under conditions of prolonged exercise, it appears that adequate mineral intake to prevent a deficiency is all that is required. See entries for each mineral for further information regarding potential influences of exercise on mineral status and mineral supplementation and performance.

Mitochondria are organelles within cells that possess the capability of producing energy from macronutrients. During exercise training, mitochondria proliferate and their function is enhanced, allowing for more energy production than during the untrained state.

Molybdenum is a micromineral that can be found in foods such as legumes, whole grains, meat, fish, and poultry. It is required for the catabolism of nucleic acids. In particular, molybdenum is needed for the function of xanthine dehydrogenase and xanthine oxidase, which are involved in purine degradation. A role for molybdenum supplementation in athletes has not been established.

Monosaccharide A monosaccharide is a single unit of a carbohydrate. The most common monosaccharides provided in the diet are glucose, fructose, and galactose.

Monounsaturated fatty acids (MUFAs) are characterized by having one double bond in their structure (as depicted in Figure M.3), which prevents them from being "saturated" with hydrogen molecules. Oleic acid, which has 18 carbons and 1 double bond is by far the most prevalent monounsaturated fatty acid in the diet.

M

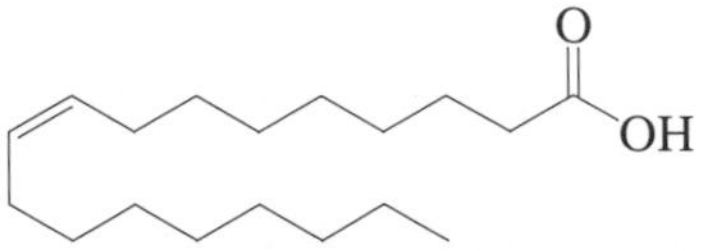

monounsaturated fatty acid (oleic acid)

FIGURE M.3

MUFAs *See* **Monounsaturated fatty acids**

Multivitamin–multimineral supplements Vitamins and minerals are needed in very small quantities for the body. Both are required for vital functions in the body, which include biochemical reactions for energy production, hemoglobin synthesis, bone health, immune function, reactions and structural properties for the synthesis and repair of muscle tissue, and the protection against oxidation processes in the body. Each vitamin and many minerals have been described in separate entries; however, some research is available regarding the effects of multivitamin–multimineral supplements on nutritional status and the performance of athletes.

Research in which the influence of a multivitamin–multimineral supplement were provided to athletes for 3 months has suggested that except for pyridoxine and riboflavin, status of the nutrients provided was unchanged.[302] The concentration of serum pyridoxine and activity of erythrocyte glutathione reductase (a marker of riboflavin status) were increased after supplementation. The authors concluded that little change occurred with intake of a multivitamin–multimineral supplement. Results of athletic performance for this study were reported in a separate paper.[303] Those experiments suggested that 3 months of multivitamin–multimineral supplementation failed to influence performance.

In similar research Telford et al. evaluated the influence of 7 to 8 months of multivitamin–multimineral supplementation on the performance of athletes participating in a variety of sports.[234] Performance was assessed in a variety of ways depending on the type of athlete. Overall, supplementation failed to produce enhancements in performance. Likewise, Singh et al. suggested that 90 days of supplementation with a similar preparation failed to influence physiological markers during a 90-minute endurance run and performance of a test to exhaustion performed immediately following the run at 90 to 100% of VO_{2max}.[233] Furthermore, isokinetic measures of strength and endurance were not affected.

These studies provide evidence suggesting that supplementation of multivitamin–multimineral mixtures is not likely to enhance performance. Furthermore, these data indirectly indicate that supplementation with any of the individual vitamins or minerals provided in these preparations is unlikely to enhance the performance of adequately nourished individuals.

Although little solid research is available regarding the dietary requirements of athletes, overall, the Dietary Reference Intakes (DRIs) established by the Food and Nutrition Board of the National Academy of Sciences appear to apply well to both athletic and nonathletic populations. However, athletes and practitioners should be aware that the nutrient requirements for some nutrients increase as energy (that is thiamin, riboflavin, niacin) or protein (such as vitamin B_6) intake increases. Furthermore, athletes that are restricting food intake, eliminating certain food groups, or consuming high carbohydrate diets with low micronutrients, seem to be in greater danger for vitamins or minerals deficiency.[213] In these cases, supplementation may be warranted; however, obtaining the necessary vitamins and minerals from foods is typically considered optimal for health and well-being.

Muscle glycogen *See* **Glycogen**

M

Muscle hyperplasia Hyperplasia of muscle cells (also called muscle fibers) is a term used to describe an increase in the number of muscle cells. Some controversy exists with regard to the contribution of hyperplasia as a result of heavy exercise. Overall, hyperplasia does not appear to be a major contributor to growth during resistance training.

Muscle hypertrophy Hypertrophy of muscle cells (also called muscle fibers) refers to the enlargement or growth of the muscle cell. Strenuous exercise can produce muscle hypertrophy, which accounts for the majority of an increase in lean body mass during resistance training. Hypertrophy occurs due to increases in the number and size of myofibrils within the muscle fiber as well as increased storage of fuels (such as triglycerides, glucose, creatine phosphate) within the cell. The development of connective tissue associated with the muscle also produces increased lean body mass during training.

Myoglobin is an iron-containing protein in muscle cells that stores and transports oxygen within the cell for exchange with carbon dioxide.

Myosin Along with actin, myosin is one of the two principal contractile proteins in the muscle cell.

N

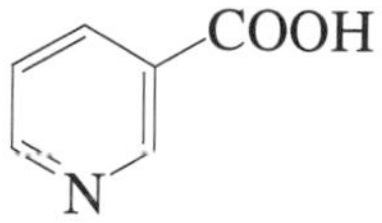

Niacin is a water-soluble vitamin available as either nicotinic acid (Figure N.1) or niacinamide (nicotinamide). Niacin has previously been known as vitamin B_3, although that title is rarely used today. Niacin typically functions in its coenzyme forms that included the oxidized and reduced forms of nicotinamide adenine dinucleotide (NAD), which are also

niacin

FIGURE N.1

needed for certain functions in their phosphorylated forms. Roles of niacin include the production of energy from macronutrients through various metabolic pathways including glycolysis, pyruvate dehydrogenase, Krebs cycle, beta-oxidation, and the electron transport system. Niacin is also needed for the synthesis of fat and glycogen.

Dietary sources of niacin include meat, fish, poultry, legumes, peanuts, peanut butter, potatoes, and enriched grains. Deficiency can produce muscular weakness and fatigue and can progress to a condition known as pellagra, which is characterized by diarrhea, dermatitis, dementia, and eventually death.

As nicotinic acid, niacin has been used for many years to lower the concentration of lipids in the blood. It appears to exert its action by inhibiting lipolysis, thereby decreasing free fatty acid mobilization into the circulation.[304,305] For this reason, when supplemented in large amounts, niacin may impair endurance exercise performance.[305,306] Therefore, niacin has been termed an ergolytic substance, rather than an ergogenic aid. However, some research has failed to detect a decrement in exercise performance.[307]

Nickel is a micromineral about which relatively little is known. Foods that provide the majority of dietary nickel often include nuts and whole grains but small amounts of nickel can be found in many foods of other food groups as well. The functions and essentiality of nickel have been difficult to establish. Potential functions include serving as a cofactor for various enzymes including urease and methlymalonlyl mutase.

Nicotinamide *See* **Niacin**

Nicotinic acid *See* **Niacin**

Nitrogen balance is used as an indicator of protein status. Each amino acid possesses nitrogen; thus, protein is the only macronutrient that provides nitrogen within the diet. When a person is in nitrogen balance, their intake of nitrogen, which is nearly all from protein, is equal to their excretion of nitrogen, which is primarily from urea, but several other sources (such as sloughed skin cells, ammonia, uric acid, creatinine, etc.) as well. Positive nitrogen balance occurs when dietary intake of nitrogen exceeds excretion. For example, an athlete who is gaining lean body mass through resistance training will be in positive balance. Negative nitrogen balance occurs when the body losses exceed dietary intake. An athlete in negative balance is losing lean body mass.

Nonessential amino acid A nonessential amino is an amino acid that can be synthesized within the body to an extent that it is not needed in the diet. Eleven nonessential amino acids (Table A.1) are required for synthesis of the body's proteins. Other nonessential amino acids that participate in biochemical reactions within the body include taurine, citrulline, and ornithine. Many amino acids that are nonessential for healthy individuals can become essential for others. For example, individuals suffering from phenylketonuria, an inborn error of phenylalanine metabolism, can eat only enough phenylalanine to provide for adequate protein synthesis; thus tyrosine becomes essential within their diet. Separate entries are provided for each nonessential amino acid.

Nonessential nutrients are substances often provided in the diet of humans that can be produced in adequate amounts within the body to meet our needs for normal growth, development, and maintenance. Dietary intake of a nonessential nutrient will decrease the demand for its production.

Nutraceutical The term nutraceutical has been used to identify food products and chemicals that potentially provide health benefits to the body aside from meeting daily requirements for normal health. Nutrients that can produce positive effects when provided at levels not usually obtainable from the diet are often considered nutraceuticals.

Nutrient A nutrient is a chemical in food that provides functions that are important for health. These may include participation in biochemical reactions, providing body structure, or contributing energy to the body. Some nutrients are essential, which means they must be provided in the diet. Other nutrients are nonessential, which means that they can be sufficiently produced within the body to meet the body's demands.

Nutrient density describes the level of a nutrient or group of nutrients in a food relative to the amount of energy provided by that food. A nutrient-dense food provides high levels of nutrients with relatively low levels of energy (Calories). A nonnutrient-dense food would provide high levels of energy with very little nutrients. Consuming a nutrient-dense diet assures an individual of meeting their daily needs with less risk of weight gain.

Nutrition can be defined in a variety of ways, but generally encompasses the oral consumption of dietary components and the utilization of nutrients within the body.

N

O

Obesity is defined as excess body weight or fatness by a variety of methods usually based on either body weight for a given height or percentage of body fatness as an indicator of overall body composition. Obesity is a growing problem in the U.S. and is an independent risk factor for a number of chronic diseases and conditions. Comprehensive reviews of factors that promote obesity and the mechanisms by which the increased risk for chronic diseases linked to obesity are beyond the scope of this book.

Optimal exercise performance for an individual is highly unlikely during periods of obesity; however, determining an ideal body weight or fatness for a given athlete is difficult if not impossible. Furthermore, body weight and fatness above norms may be beneficial for some sports such as wrestling, sumo wrestling, and certain positions in football.

Octacosanol is a 28-carbon alcohol sometimes referred to as octacosyl alcohol. It is a component of wax extracted from plants such as wheat germ, from which it is typically available as part of a mixture called policosanol. Although there is no known biological need for octacosanol, it has been marketed as an ergogenic aid and may have cholesterol-lowering effects and provide cytoprotective and antiaggregatory properties. There is little research available for assessing its ergogenic potential. A recent review indicates that supplementation with 1 mg of octacosanol may improve reaction time and grip strength in humans and that maximal oxygen consumption is improved in patients with cardiovascular disease after consumption of 5 mg of policosanol twice per day for 20 months.[308]

Omega-3 fatty acids possess their first double bond on the third carbon from the methyl group end of the hydrocarbon chain. Alpha-linolenic acid (ALA) is an omega-3 fatty acid that is essential in the diet. Other particularly important polyunsaturated fatty acids (PUFAs) in the diet are eicosapentaenoic acid (EPA) and docosahexaenoic acid (DHA). Consumption of EPA and DHA can reduce the need for ALA consumption.

Eicosanoids are compounds that have hormone-like effects and are synthesized by cyclooxygenase and lipoxygenase enzyme systems from long-chain fatty acids such as ALA, EPA, and DHA as well as

O

129

nonomega-3 fatty acids. Eicosanoid compounds include thromboxanes, leukotrienes, and prostaglandins. The functions and potencies
of eicosanoids vary both among classifications and within each group
depending upon which fatty acid is used for its synthesis. Functions
of various eicosanoids include blood vessel or bronchiole dilation or
constriction, platelet aggregation or antiaggregation, pro- or antiinflammatory responses, chemotaxis, and other roles.

Eicosanoids produced from omega-3 fatty acids generally produce
more favorable metabolic effects than those produced from omega-6
and omega-9 fatty acids. Due to their positive metabolic effects, such
as vasodilation and reduced platelet aggregation, thereby allowing
increased blood flow and oxygen delivery to tissues, these eicosanoids
have been theorized to produce ergogenic benefits in endurance athletes. However, no available studies have directly administered
eicosanoids to determine if they provide a true ergogenic benefit.

Some researchers have fed foods rich in omega-3 fatty acids and
assessed potential benefits with no indication of an ergogenic effect.
In one study 5.2 g of fish oil containing 1.60 g of eicosapentaenoic
acid and 1.04 g of docosahexaenoic acid (both omega-3 fatty acids)
were fed to male soccer players daily for 10 weeks.[309] Maximal
aerobic power, anaerobic power, and running performance were not
improved in comparison to corn oil supplementation. Furthermore,
doses of 6 g of fish oil per day failed to enhance endurance after
3 weeks of supplementation in trained cyclists.[310]

Omega-6 fatty acids have their first double bond on the sixth carbon of the
hydrocarbon chain when counting from the methyl end of the fatty
acid. The primary dietary omega-6 fatty acid is linoleic acid, which
is an essential fatty acid since humans lack the necessary enzyme to
synthesize it. Arachidonic acid, which is supplied only in small
amounts within the diet, is of great importance for metabolism, but
may be synthesized from linoleic acid. Arachnidonic acid is particularly important for the production of various eicosanoids, which have
been described in a separate entry.

Oral rehydration *See* **Hydration status**

Organic foods Foods grown with natural pesticides and fertilizers vs. those
extracted or synthesized by man are considered to be organically
grown.

Ornithine Ornithine is a nonessential amino acid synthesized from arginine.
It is not utilized for the production of proteins but is integral in the
urea cycle for the catabolism of amino acids and elimination of nitrogen from the body.

Ornithine, also available as the supplement ornitihine-alpha-keto-glutarate, has been marketed as an ergogenic aid through its purported ability to increase levels of human growth hormone, thereby enhancing production of muscle. As reviewed by Williams, most available research does not support a role for ornithine supplementation in raising growth hormone concentration.[289] As described in the entry for growth hormone, even direct injections of growth hormone are unlikely to enhance muscle synthesis in those who produce adequate levels endogenously.

Osmolality is the concentration of particles in a solution and determines the pressure that is exerted across a membrane. Osmolality is expressed as the moles of a solute per kilogram of solvent. Osmolarity also describes the particles in a solution, but is expressed in terms of liters of solution rather than by weight.

Osteoporosis literally means porous bone and occurs when bone loses its mineral mass (bone mineral content or BMC) and calcium concentration (bone mineral density or BMD) and progressively becomes brittle. It affects 25 million individuals in the U.S., 80 to 90% of whom are women, and causes 1.5 million fractures each year; among women over 60 years of age, this disease has reached almost epidemic proportions.[73] Bone tissue is very dynamic in that it constantly undergoes cycles of resorption and deposition. Normally, peak bone mass is achieved between the ages of 18 and 25 years.[71] After peak bone mass is reached, both men and women lose bone at a rate of 0.3 to 0.5% per year.[227] At menopause, women experience an approximately 3% per year bone decline in bone mass for an average of 10 years, after which it returns to a rate of about 0.3% per year. The increased rate of bone loss during these years occurs as a result of lack of estrogen and subsequent bone resorption.

Normal BMD is often defined as that which is above the mean or less than 1.0 standard deviation (SD) below the mean for a particular age group and gender. Criteria for osteoporosis often includes a BMD greater than 2.5 SD below the mean, while osteopenia is defined as BMD between 1.0 to 2.5 SD below the mean. Risk factors of osteoporosis include being a white or Asian woman, having a sedentary lifestyle, early menopause, excess sodium intake, alcohol abuse, cigarette smoking, family history, and calcium and vitamin D deficiency.[73]

Previously thought to be a disorder of elderly women, it is now clear that young female athletes are also at risk. Premature bone loss and inadequate bone formation can also occur, resulting in low bone mineral density, increased skeletal fragility, and increased risk for

O

stress fractures of the extremities, hip, and spine.[225] Women with amenorrhea (both athletes and nonathletes) have been shown to have lower vertebral bone mineral densities compared with healthy women.[227] The prevalence of amenorrhea among female athletes ranges between 3 to 66% (depending on the population studied).[229] The skeletal status of these young women depends on the length and severity of their menstrual disturbance, the type of skeletal loading prior to the onset of amenorrhea, nutritional status, and genetic factors.[203] Research in the past 10 years has demonstrated that the premature osteoporosis in women with amenorrhea is partially irreversible even after resumption of menses, estrogen replacement, or calcium supplementation.[225,227] Osteoporosis in young athletes can result in a bone mass loss of 2 to 6% per year, with the complete loss reaching approximately 25% of the total bone mass. If unchecked, a young athlete may develop the bone mass of a 60-year-old woman, which puts her at a threefold risk of stress fractures.[227]

It is imperative that young female athletes consume adequate dietary energy to prevent amenorrhea during training. Furthermore, all athletes should ensure that daily calcium needs are being met.

Overload principle The overload principle states that muscle growth will not occur unless the muscle is stressed at a level beyond normal loads. Thus, for resistance training to be effective in increasing lean body mass, the exercises performed must provide an adequate threshold of resistance before significant growth will occur.

Overtraining syndrome is not well understood, but occurs in times of excess training with inadequate recovery and often includes nontraining stressors. Overtraining can produce a variety of symptoms, which include poor athletic performance, depressed immune function, altered mood states, weight loss, muscle pain, and overuse injuries. The most effective treatment for overtraining is rest. Recovery may take several weeks or even months depending on the severity of the condition. A less severe form of overtraining has been termed overreaching, which usually requires less time for recovery.[311]

The nutrient most studied with regard to potential implications in alleviating overtraining or overreaching is glutamine. Plasma glutamine concentrations typically fall with prolonged endurance exercise. In overtrained individuals, the concentration of plasma glutamine and the ratio of plasma glutamine to glutamate have been observed to be depressed. Some research suggests that glutamine supplementation can improve markers of immune function and even decrease risk of infection, while other studies have not produced similar results.[312] Future research to more conclusively address the metabolic responses to overtraining and the potential role of glutamine in preventing or treating overtraining is needed.

Overweight can be defined in many ways, but is simply a body weight in excess of a weight considered to be healthy but below a weight considered obese. Comprehensive reviews of factors that promote the development of excess weight as well as the mechanisms by which being overweight increases risk for chronic diseases are beyond the scope of this book.

Optimal exercise performance for an individual is highly unlikely during periods of overweight; however, determining an ideal body weight or fatness for a given athlete is difficult if not impossible. Furthermore, body weight and fatness above norms may be beneficial for some sports such as wrestling, sumo wrestling, and certain positions in football.

Ovolactovegetarian *See* **Lactoovovegeterian**

Ovovegetarian An ovovegetarian will consume eggs in addition to plant foods, but will not consume meat, fish, poultry, or dairy foods.

O

P

Pangamic acid   is a substance commonly marketed as vitamin B_{15} or dimethylglycine. Its actual identity in some preparations is not clear, since many chemicals have been marketed as pangamic acid or vitamin B15. As reviewed by Antonio and Stout, well-designed studies do not support the use of pangamic acid as an ergogenic aid.[313]

Pantothenic acid (Figure P.1) is a water-soluble vitamin distributed in a large variety of foods within the diet. Its primary functions are serving as part of coenzyme A as well as acyl carrier protein, which is involved in fatty acid synthesis.

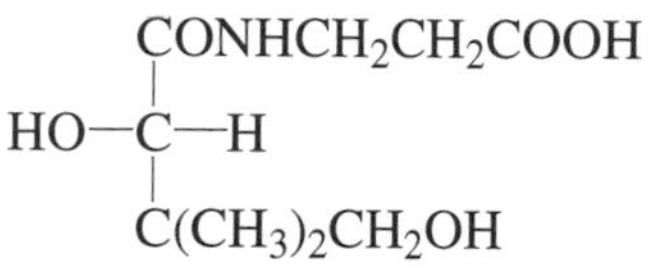

$$CONHCH_2CH_2COOH$$
$$HO-C-H$$
$$C(CH_3)_2CH_2OH$$

pantothenic acid

FIGURE P.1

The vast majority of research examining a potential role of pantothenic acid in improving athletic performance has not demonstrated such effects. In one study, the effects of a pantothenic acid and thiamin supplementation were assessed in trained cyclists. The cyclists consumed 1 g of allithiamin and 1.8 g of a pantethine/ pantothenic acid mixture for 7 days prior to testing of exercise metabolism and performance. No differences in performance, blood concentrations of lactate, glucose, or free fatty acids, or other physiological measures were detected in comparison to a placebo.[314] In another study, supplementation of 1 g of pantothenic acid for 2 weeks did not improve performance in trained runners.[315] Furthermore, multivitamin–multimineral preparations containing panthenic acid have failed to enhance performance.[67,68,303]

Peptide   A peptide is more than one amino acid linked together by a peptide bond. A dipeptide contains two amino acids, while a tripeptide contains three. Polypeptides are often defined as having more than three peptides. Some references consider a polypeptide to have up to 100 amino acids, while others limit the definition to only 50. Molecules with greater than these numbers of amino acids linked by peptide bonds are considered proteins. The potential metabolic influences of certain short peptides found in foods or produced from proteins during the digestive process is beginning to receive much attention in research

135

and may some day prove to have implications for health or performance of athletes.

Pesticides are chemicals used to kill insects while growing food. Pesticides currently available in the U.S. are considered safe for use as long as the food is adequately washed before preparation and consumption.

Phenylalanine (Figure P.2) is an essential amino acid involved in protein structure as well as many nonprotein functions. Phenylalanine is used to produce tyrosine, which can subsequently be metabolized to a variety of neurotransimitters and hormones including L-DOPA, dopamine, norepinephrine, epinephrine, melanin, and thyroid hormone. Potential ergogenic roles of phenylalanine have not been identified.

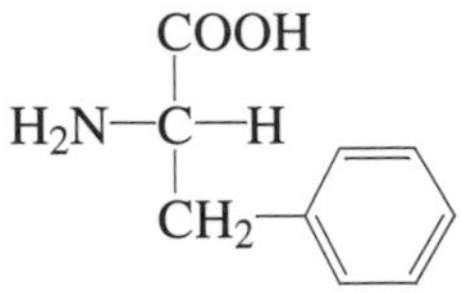

phenylalanine

FIGURE P.2

Phosphagens are compounds that possess a high-energy phosphate bond that when broken produces energy that can be used to drive biochemical reactions such as muscle contraction, active transport, and biosynthesis. Adenosine triphosphate (ATP) is most commonly used for these purposes within the body. Another important phosphagen is creatine phosphate, which is used extensively to restore ATP levels during strenuous activity.

Phosphate salts of sodium and potassium have been proposed to be ergogenic for several reasons. Proposed mechanisms include increased availability of phosphate for oxidative phosphorylation and phosphocreatine synthesis, production of 2,3-diphosphoglycerate, which is important for delivery of oxygen to tissues via hemoglobin, and buffering the accumulation of hydrogen ions in the blood, thus maintaining a lower pH.

Ergogenic benefits of supplementation have been observed in some studies, while other studies have not supported these effects. Doses of supplements ranging from approximately 1 to 5 g of phosphate salts have typically been studied and periods of supplementation have typically ranged from 1 to 6 days. Results have indicated either enhanced performance of endurance exercise[316–319] or no changes or differences in performance.[320,321] The studies demonstrating improved running and cycling performance utilized a dosing regimen of 1 g of sodium phosphate 4 times each day for 3 to 6 days. Since few overall studies have been conducted on these compounds and the findings vary, future research is typically recommended by experts in the field. However, since detecting differences in athletic performance is often difficult, phosphate salts hold great promise as a means to enhance endurance in some situations.

Concern that excess consumption of phosphate salts can impair calcium balance exists. The extent that the use of phosphate salts for athletic performance could alter bone health has not been investigated; however, research into this possibility is warranted.

Phosphocreatine *See* **Creatine**

Phospholipids belong to a large family of molecules containing both lipid and phosphate components (such as glycerophosphatides, sphingolipids, etc.). In particular, glycerophosphatides (Figure P.3) consist of a glycerol bound to two fatty acids and a phosphate molecule that is linked to one of many compounds including choline, serine, ethanolamine, and inositol. Phosphatidyl choline, also known as lecithin, is a primary example of a phospholipid. The functions of phospholipids include serving as a major constituent of cell membranes, participating in biochemical reactions, and as an important structural and functional component of tissues of the central and peripheral nervous systems.

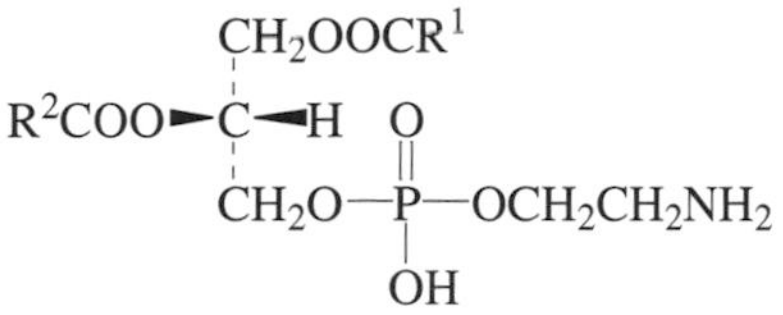

$$CH_2OOCR^1$$
$$R^2COO\!-\!C\!-\!H \quad O$$
$$CH_2O\!-\!\overset{\|}{P}\!-\!OCH_2CH_2NH_2$$
$$OH$$

phospholipid

FIGURE P.3

Phosphorus is a macromineral that serves many critical functions in the body. Dietary phosphorus can be provided by a wide range of foods including meat, fish, poultry, dairy foods, eggs, legumes, grains, and nuts. Many of the functions that phosphorus serves are related to its roles in the structural properties of important compounds. Much of the crystalline structure of bone includes phosphorus. It is also an important structural component of cell membranes, which require phosphorus for the production of phospholipids. Phosphate molecules also produce the high-energy bonds of chemicals such as adenosine triphosphate, creatine phosphate, and others. Coenzyme forms of many vitamins (such as thiamin, riboflavin, niacin, and vitamin B_6) also require phosphate.

Although deficiency of phosphorus is rare, given its availability in many foods, without adequate dietary phosphorus muscular weakness and impaired bone health are probable symptoms. Many phosphorus-containing supplements have been used to potentially improve performance. While some do not appear to be effective (such as ATP supplements), others appear to be of potential use for specific types of exercise.

Most notably, creatine and creatine phosphate supplements have been demonstrated to enhance muscle creatine phosphate concentrations and improve performance of repetitive bouts of exercise performed at high levels of intensity. See the entry for creatine for a thorough description of its ergogenic effects and limitations.

Phosphate salts have also been studied for their potential role in enhancing performance. Although some studies have detected no improvements in performance following supplementation, others have reported improvements of physiological responses to exercise as well as enhanced performance. The most often cited mechanism for improved performance is increased levels of 2,3-diphosphoglycerate, which can improve oxygen dissociation for more effective delivery to tissues. The entry on phosphate salts provides more information on their supplementation and exercise performance effects.

Phylloquinone *See* **Vitamin K**

Phytochemicals are chemicals found in plants that may offer benefits to health. Many phytochemicals available from foods are also considered phytonutrients. These chemicals provide an assortment of potential functions and often include antioxidant or estrogenic activity. Many phytochemicals have been studied for potential performance-enhancing capabilities and more research is underway.

Placebo In sport nutrition a placebo is an inert compound provided in a separate trial or to a separate study group to ensure that research findings are not the result of a placebo effect, but rather the results of the experimental compound being tested. A placebo effect occurs when the suggestive powers of experimentation produce a physiological or physical response.

Polysaccharide A polysaccharide is a carbohydrate containing more than two monosaccharides linked by glycosidic bonds. The most common polysaccharides provided in the diet are amylose and amylopectin, which are often collectively referred to as starches.

Polyunsaturated fatty acids (PUFAs) are characterized by having more than one double bond in their structure, which prevents them from being "saturated" with hydrogen molecules (see Figure P.4). Linoleic and linolenic acids are the most common PUFAs in the diet. Alpha-linolenic acid (ALA) and linoleic acid are essential fatty acids. Other particularly important PUFAs in the diet are eicosapentaenoic acid

(EPA) and docosahexaenoic acid (DHA). Along with ALA, these are the predominant omega-3 fatty acids in the diet. Linoleic acid is the most common omega-6 fatty acid in the diet. An important omega-6 fatty acid in metabolism, but not eaten in large quantities, is arachidonic acid. See the entries for fatty acids, essential fatty acids, omega-3 fatty acids, and omega-6 fatty acids for more information about polyunsaturated fatty acids.

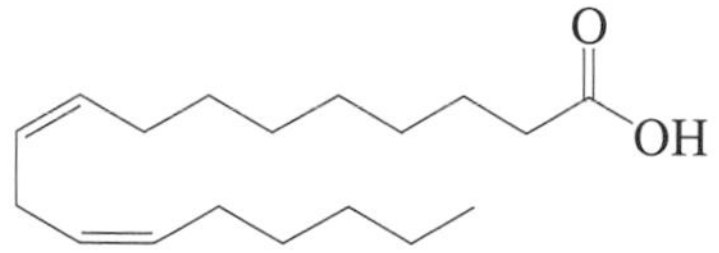

polyunsaturated fatty acid (linoleic acid)

FIGURE P.4

Postexercise nutrition Proper nutrition after exercise can be extremely important, especially following vigorous training sessions or for events that take place on consecutive days. For endurance athletes, the primary goal for postexercise nutrition is to replace lost glycogen stores, while for resistance training the goal is to promote protein synthesis to maintain or enhance lean body mass. Details regarding postexercise recommendations for glycogen resynthesis are provided in the carbohydrate entry. Some research suggests that protein consumption following resistance training may be important for maximizing body protein synthesis. This concept is discussed more completely in the entry for protein.

Potassium is a macromineral found within the body as the most predominant intracellular cation. In the diet, potassium is obtained from an array of fresh foods including fruits (such as bananas, citrus fruits, peaches, and more), vegetables (such as potatoes, broccoli, etc.), dairy foods, and eggs. Potassium is critical for electrolyte balance, which controls, at least to some extent, fluid balance, action potentials/nerve transmission, active transport mechanisms, and more. Adequate intake of potassium appears to be important for the prevention of hypertension. Deficiency of potassium can also produce muscular weakness and cardiac arrhythmias when blood levels drop below normal, a condition referred to as hypokalemia. The importance of potassium with regard to electrolyte replacement in athletes is discussed in the entry for electrolytes.

Precompetition nutrition *See* **Preevent meal**

Preevent meal Many athletes focus on proper food consumption in the hours and moments just prior to exercise or competition. Williams has outlined several guidelines that should be used by athletes during the meal prior to competition.[96] These recommendations include consumption of a meal providing foods that will allow the stomach to be relatively empty before the event. The meal should be high in carbohydrate and relatively low in fiber, fat, and protein. It should usually be eaten approximately 3 to 4 hours before competition to allow for stomach emptying and nutrient utilization. Liquid meals are often less likely to cause gastrointestinal disturbances (such as cramps, gas, nausea, diarrhea) and may be consumed closer to the event (that is 2 to 3 hours prior). As described in the entry for liquid meals, consumption of a liquid meal may be the optimal choice for early morning events that begin relatively soon after waking. Personal preferences based on taste, adequate energy and water content, and absence of gastrointestinal disturbances, should be the major factors in determining what is consumed for a preevent meal. Many commercial products provide the benefit of convenience; however, there are no magical foods or products that will improve the performance of all athletes. Although a good pregame meal can not replace good overall dietary habits, it can remain an important part of performance enhancement and contribute to adequate daily intake of nutrients.

Proline (Figure P.5) is a nonessential amino acid used in the formation of the body's proteins. It is particularly important, along with vitamin C, for the synthesis of collagen. Potential ergogenic roles of proline have not been identified.

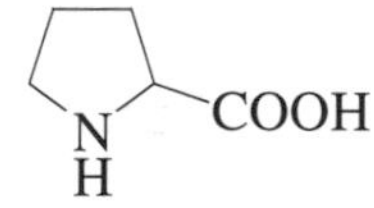

proline

FIGURE P.5

Proteins are characterized by many amino acids linked together by peptide bonds. Proteins are often defined as having at least 50 amino acids, while others suggest that at least 100 amino acids are needed for a molecule to be considered a protein. Those molecules with less amino acids in their structures are considered polypeptides. Foods rich in protein include meat, fish, poultry, eggs, legumes, diary foods, and others. Protein is also found in nuts, seeds, grains, and vegetables, while very little is present in fruits. Protein is needed in the diet because it provides essential amino acids, which are described in a separate entry.

Dietary proteins include 20 amino acids in their structures. Nine of these amino acids are considered essential. The functions of the amino acids vary from one to another and are described in separate entries for each individual amino acid. One common function of each of these 20 amino acids is the production of the body's proteins, which include structural proteins, enzymes, hormones, immunoglobulins, transport proteins, and storage proteins.

Research suggests that athletes require consumption of more protein than nonathletes.[322] The dietary recommendation for protein for the average healthy adult is to consume 0.8 g protein for each kilogram of body weight. Typically, research indicates that strength-trained athletes should consume in the range of 1.5 to 1.7 g per kg of body weight and that endurance athletes require 1.2 to 1.6 g per kg of body weight.[322] While this is a substantially higher protein requirement, average, nonathletic Americans consume within these ranges of intake as part of their usual diets.[323] Since athletes who are not on a weight loss diet require a greater daily intake of energy for normal weight balance, this group rarely has difficulty obtaining their dietary needs of protein from regular food. Regardless, many athletes believe that they need extremely large quantities of protein and find protein-rich beverages and sports bars to be convenient sources of protein.

Athletes most often concerned about their protein intake are those who use resistance training for their sport. To date, however, relatively little research has evaluated the efficacy of protein feeding following resistance/weight training on protein synthesis or lean body mass development. One study suggested that in older men protein feeding after exercise can enhance muscle growth and some but not all measures of strength.[324] In that study, 13 men were fed 10 g of protein, 7 g of carbohydrate, and 3 g of fat in a liquid preparation immediately or 2 hours after resistance exercise performed 3 times per week for 12 weeks. Improvements in muscle growth and strength were apparent when protein was eaten immediately after exercise but not when eaten 2 hours after. Research has also demonstrated that consumption of carbohydrate and essential amino acids[325] or carbohydrate, whey protein, and amino acids[326] after exercise improves muscle protein synthesis. Furthermore, one study has indicated that ingestion of essential amino acids with carbohydrate prior to exercise may provide greater benefits for muscle protein synthesis in comparison to feedings immediately after exercise.[327]

Other research has demonstrated that feeding protein after resistance exercise can positively alter the hormone levels in the blood in a way that may enhance body protein synthesis.[328] Although this is not direct evidence that increases in muscle can occur, it does provide some additional evidence for the possibility. Various proteins and protein products including nonanimal sources have been demonstrated to have this effect. In two studies, wheat protein hydrolysate (along with the amino acids leucine and phenylalanine) raised plasma insulin levels, which may promote body protein synthesis.[329,330] Other researchers have observed similar responses with unreported whole

P

protein sources.[331] Researchers have noted that the phenomena may be related to the total energy (calories) fed following exercise, rather than protein itself. Additionally, some research suggests that protein fed along with carbohydrate can improve synthesis of muscle glycogen (carbohydrate stores), which has potential implications for recovery that may promote increased ability to carry out subsequent exercise training.[329,332]

The type of protein consumed may have effects on the outcomes of training. Few studies, however, have been conducted to determine if weight trainers or bodybuilders can synthesize more muscle from the consumption of one particular protein than another. Some research has suggested that older men consuming diets containing protein predominantly from either beef or lactoovovegetarian sources had no differences in change in muscle size or strength during resistance training.[333] In other research, two studies have reported that casein may be used preferentially for body protein synthesis when compared to whey.[334,335] For both of the studies, the two proteins were fed to subjects at rest on separate occasions following overnight fasts. Over several hours, blood and breath collections revealed that whey protein was digested and absorbed more rapidly and was more likely to be metabolized for energy than casein and that casein was more likely to be used for protein synthesis. These studies did not demonstrate which proteins of the body were being synthesized nor did they address the issue of changes in body musculature during times of bodybuilding. Along with the previously described research, these results provide investigators with a potential reason to conduct such studies to determine if some proteins are better than others when fed at particular times relative to training. No other proteins have been similarly compared, which makes it impossible to assess the efficacy of other proteins (such as egg, soy, etc.) in comparison to whey or casein.

Recently, researchers have addressed the implications of protein consumption on exercise metabolism and performance during endurance activities. Although research is needed to explore the possible benefits in more detail, results to date have suggested some promising effects. For example, when protein was fed along with carbohydrate during intermittent endurance exercise, time to exhaustion was extended in comparison to carbohydrate feeding alone.[103] This study has been criticized, since the energy contents between the feedings differed slightly, which may at least partially account for the differences in performance. However, in one study a feeding of carbohydrate and protein produced enhanced performance compared to an isocaloric feeding including carbohydrate only.[336]

Overall, adequate dietary protein intake is essential for both endurance and resistance-training athletes. Although requirements are somewhat higher than for nonathletes, obtaining adequate protein is rather easy. New research suggests that protein timing may affect synthesis of protein and glycogen following exercise and that protein incorporated into a sports drink may be of benefit to endurance exercisers.

Protein powders are used in drink mixes to provide supplementary protein to the diet. Many preparations of protein powders have been developed and often include whole milk proteins, whey protein, casein, soy protein, egg albumin, and combinations of these. Although drinks produced from protein powders can offer a convenient source of protein and essential amino acids, research has not demonstrated their efficacy over whole foods in the development of lean body mass in exercisers. The entry for proteins provides more detail regarding the protein needs of athletes.

Protein-sparing Sparing of body protein is important for maintenance of lean body mass. Adequate energy and protein intake are vital to prevent catabolism of lean tissue. Dietary carbohydrate is well known for its protein-sparing effects. Sparing protein is of particular importance for an athlete during periods of weight loss, in which maintenance of lean body mass is difficult. When energy intake is restricted, adequate protein intake becomes essential to preserve as much lean tissue as possible. During weight loss, the dietary protein requirement when expressed as a percentage of energy intake climbs as the degree of restriction increases.

PUFAs *See* **Polyunsaturated fatty acids**

Pycnogenol is an extract from French maritime pine bark (Pinus maritima), and is considered to be a strong and direct antioxidant and therefore is used as a dietary supplement. Pycnogenol is claimed to alleviate inflammations, improve cardiovascular function, inhibit tumor initiation, and inhibit angiotensin-conversion enzyme. It has been suggested to take part in the prevention of some degenerative diseases such as diabetes, cancer, and atherosclerosis due to its ability to protect body cells from damage by reactive oxygen and nitrogen.[337] No studies are available to support ergogenic or health benefits in athletes.

Pyridoxine *See* **Vitamin B$_6$**

Pyruvate *See* **Pyruvic acid**

Pyruvate dehydrogenase complex The pyruvate dehydrogenase complex is responsible for converting pyruvate to acetyl CoA in the cytosol of a cell. When pyruvate is produced from glucose during glycolysis, for further metabolism via Krebs cycle, it must first be converted to acetyl CoA. The pyruvate dehydrogenase complex requires many enzymes and cofactors to accomplish this reaction. Cofactors involved include coenzyme A, which includes pantothenic acid as part of its structure, NAD^+ (coenzyme form of niacin), FAD (coenzyme form of riboflavin), and TDP (coenzyme form of thiamin), as well as magnesium and lipoic acid. During the series of reactions, carbon dioxide is eliminated and $NADH + H^+$ is produced, which can be used for ATP synthesis through the electron transport system.

Pyruvic acid (Figure P.6), also known as pyruvate, is a 3-carbon intermediate of metabolism produced primarily via aerobic glycolysis from glucose and from the transamination of alanine. Although the functions of pyruvate are varied, a principal use of pyruvate is for energy production through the pyruvate dehydrogenase complex, which produces acetyl CoA and $NADH + H^+$ and elimination of carbon dioxide. The acetyl CoA produced can then enter Krebs cycle, which yields molecules that along with the $NADH + H^+$ formed in the pyruvate dehydrogenase complex can produce ATP through the electron transport system.

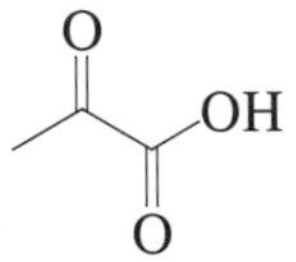

pyruvic acid

FIGURE P.6

Since pyruvate is used for the production of energy, its potential as an ergogenic aid has been examined, but only to a limited extent. Research suggests that doses of 7 g of pyruvate per day are ineffective in enhancing endurance.[338] However, when pyruvate was supplemented at very high doses (25 g) combined with 75 g of another important metabolic intermediate (dihydroxacetone) for 7 days, it improved endurance in both arm ergometry and cycling ergometry to fatigue.[339,340] It is unclear if pyruvate could enhance endurance under similar situations if supplemented alone and the threshold that is required to obtain similar results. Consuming pyruvate and dihydroxyacetone at these levels is not practical and would be extremely expensive.

Pyruvate has also been studied for potential influences on body composition. Research suggests that pyruvate at relatively high doses (at least 6 g per day) may be effective in producing weight loss.[341] That study has been criticized for several issues including no weight loss exhibited by the placebo and control groups, which like the experimental group were allowed limited (2000 kcal) energy consumption and participated in a moderate exercise program expected to produce weight loss.[342] Furthermore, more women were in the experimental group receiving pyruvate than in the placebo and control groups.

P

Q

Quackery Nutritional quackery includes the sale or promotion of questionable and sometimes harmful products purported to have positive health or performance effects using misleading tactics. New products are continually made available to consumers such as athletes. It is often difficult for the consumer to discern a questionable product from one that is legitimate. In the case of ergogenic prospects, athletes and practitioners should consider the following simple tips when evaluating the claims.

1. Determine if the claims made seem too good to be true. Unbelievable claims are almost always a sign of quackery.
2. Do not accept testimonials as fact, even when they come from successful athletes. While the testimonial may be based on the true feelings of an athlete, many factors can mislead an individual into believing that a product is working for them. Consumers must also be aware that an athlete endorsing a product may be biased.
3. An athlete, coach, or athletic trainer should seek the advice of a registered dietitian if the legitimacy of a product is unclear.

The National Council Against Health Fraud (NCAHF) is a reliable source of information about questionable products. Furthermore, published guidelines and Internet Web sites of organizations providing evidence-based information such as the American Dietetic Association and its practice group called Sports, Cardiovascular and Wellness Nutritionists, the American College of Sports Medicine, the American Society for Nutritional Sciences, and the American Medical Association can be very useful for current nutritional information. Government organizations such as the Food and Drug Administration, the Department of Health and Human Services, and the National Institutes of Health can also be valuable sources of reliable information.

R

Ratings of perceived exertion are commonly used to gauge the perceived level of effort that is experienced by an exercising individual. The most common such scales range from either 6 through 20 or 1 through 10. Each scale provides descriptors corresponding to the level of difficulty as perceived by the individual. These ratings are commonly used in sports nutrition research to assess the efficacy of a dietary technique or supplement in enhancing performance. Although this is not a direct indicator of performance, it can be useful for providing evidence of a potential ergogenic capacity and can suggest that more research is needed to confirm an ergogenic benefit.

RDA *See* **Recommended Dietary Allowance**

RDIs *See* **Reference Daily Intakes**

Reactive hypoglycemia is a transient form of hypoglycemia that occurs in response to consumption of a carbohydrate-rich meal or food followed by vigorous exercise, usually about 15 to 60 minutes later. After consumption of the meal, blood glucose concentration rises, which stimulates the secretion of insulin from the pancreas. Insulin is a potent hormone that produces a decrease in blood glucose concentration. While insulin is carrying out its function, the subsequent exercise also enhances tissue uptake of glucose. The result is a transient hypoglycemia, which can lead to the sensation of fatigue and thus impair exercise performance of some athletes. While this has been demonstrated in some research,[276] many other studies have failed to detect either hypoglycemia or impaired endurance performance with similar protocols. As described in the entry for glycemic index, some but not all research suggests that feedings of lower glycemic index foods may be optimal as preexercise feedings within this time frame.

RD *See* **Registered dietitian**

Recommended Dietary Allowance (RDA) The Recommended Dietary Allowances is one of four possible Dietary Reference Intake (DRI) values established by the Food and Nutrition Board of the National Academy of Sciences. The RDA is defined as the average daily intake level that is sufficient to meet the nutrient needs of nearly all (97.5%) healthy individuals within a certain age range and gender.

Reference Daily Intakes (RDIs) The Reference Daily Intakes are a set of dietary references based on the Dietary Reference Intake value (either

Recommended Dietary Allowances or Adequate Intake values) for essential vitamins and minerals. These values are used in food labeling to allow consumers to gauge the nutrient content of a serving of a particular food item.

Registered dietitian (RD) A registered dietitian is the premiere provider of health care related to nutrition and foods in the U.S. RDs receive their credential by the Commission on Dietetic Registration, the credentialing agency for the American Dietetic Association. Registered dietitians are comprehensively educated and trained in the ability to translate scientific information into appropriate food choices and to provide medical nutrition therapy. Athletes, coaches, athletic trainers, and others should consult a registered dietitian when seeking nutritional advice and counseling for sports performance. Many registered dietitians who work with athletes are members of the Sports, Cardiovascular and Wellness Nutritionists (SCAN) dietetic practice group of the American Dietetic Association, which can be contacted at www.scandpg.org.

Respiratory exchange ratio (R or RER) The respiratory exchange ratio is assessed through assessment of expired gases as the volume of carbon dioxide produced divided by the volume of oxygen consumed. RER provides an indication of the respiratory quotient (RQ), which describes the ratio of metabolic gas exchange at the level of the cell. RQ gives an indication of the mixture of fuels utilized for energy at rest or during a specific task. In general, as RQ approaches 1.00, carbohydrate is providing a larger percentage of fuel for metabolism. Conversely, as RQ approaches 0.70, fat is providing a larger percentage of fuel being utilized. The RQ of protein is typically about 0.82 but is not assessed by exhaled gases.

During exercise, protein typically provides a relatively small percentage of the fuel catabolized for energy. As exercise intensity increases, carbohydrate utilization increases at an absolute rate and as a percentage of energy expenditure; thus, RQ and RER increase as well.

Respiratory quotient *See* **Respiratory exchange ratio**

Retinol *See* **Vitamin A**

Riboflavin (see Figure R.1), also known as vitamin B_2, is a water-soluble vitamin that functions in oxidation–reduction reactions in either the reduced or oxidized form of flavin mononucleotide (FMN) or flavin adenine dinucleotide (FAD). Riboflavin is particularly important in biochemical reactions that allow the production of energy from food. Metabolic pathways that require riboflavin include beta-oxidation, the pyruvate dehydrogenase complex, Krebs cycle, and the electron

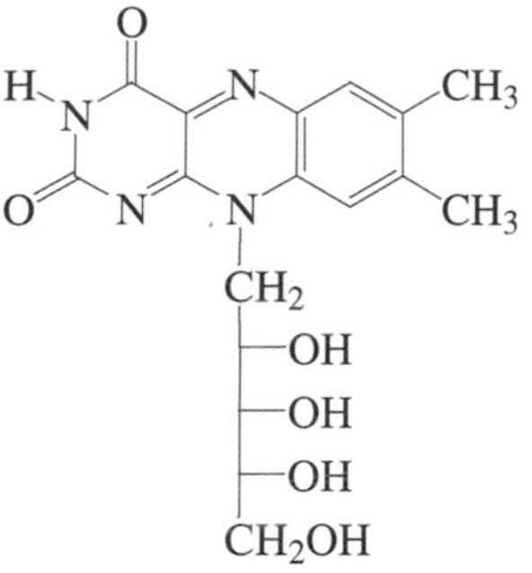

riboflavin (vitamin B$_2$)

FIGURE R.1

transport system. Foods rich in riboflavin include meat, fish, poultry, dairy products, whole and enriched grains, and leafy, green vegetables.

Exercise may lower riboflavin status somewhat[343–345]; however, riboflavin supplementation does not appear to enhance exercise performance. Supplementation of 10 mg per day has been demonstrated to lower neuromuscular irritability,[346] but this effect does not necessarily translate to improved endurance. Overall, since training may decrease status, supplementation may eventually prove to be beneficial in preventing decreased performance in those who begin an exercise program in a deficient or near-deficient state; however, currently available research has not confirmed this possibility, even when supplementation enhances status.[302,303]

Ribose (Figure R.2) is a 5-carbon sugar produced from glucose for the synthesis of nucleotides. Recently, several studies have examined the effect of ribose on adenosine triphosphate (ATP) formation and performance in athletes. To date, research has failed to demonstrate that ribose supplementation improves performance of activities performed at high intensities.[347–350] Results are split regarding the efficacy of supplementation to produce higher concentrations of ATP in the muscle. One study suggests that ATP levels are enhanced,[347] while another has detected no effect.[348] Overall, the available data do not warrant ribose supplementation for performance enhancement.

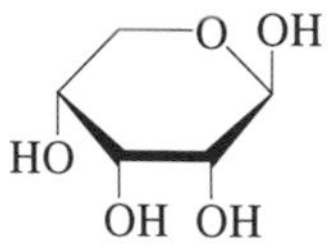

ribose

FIGURE R.2

S

Saccharide The term saccharide means sugar or sweet and is often used as a synonym for carbohydrate.

Salt tablets Although salt tablets are not as popular today as they have been in the past, some athletes still use them to replenish lost electrolytes and the organizers of some prolonged adventure races require their possession by competitors. The entry for electrolytes describes their importance for prolonged exercise; however, salt tablets are generally not considered necessary for competition. During prolonged events or training sessions, particularly in hot or humid climates, fluid and sodium loss can be great. If plain water is provided for fluid replacement throughout the exercise period, hyponatremia can develop. Although salt tablets may be effective in replacing the lost sodium, most researchers suggest consumption of a beverage containing electrolytes for their replacement.

S-adenosylmethionine (SAM-e) is considered a chief physiological methyl donor.[351] SAM-e manufacturers claim that it is beneficial for treating a wide range of ailments including depression, osteoarthritis, liver disease, multiple sclerosis, Parkinson's disease, and migraine headaches. There are no known benefits of SAM-e supplementation for athletes.

Saturated fatty acids Fatty acids are commonly classified based on their degree of saturation with hydrogen atoms, which is determined by the absence or presence of double bonds between carbon atoms. Saturated fatty acids have no double bonds and are therefore "saturated" with hydrogen ions as depicted by the example in Figure S.1.

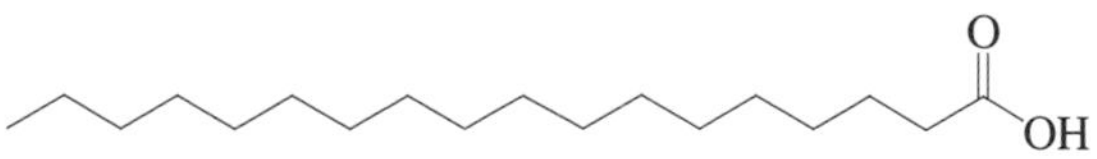

saturated fatty acid (stearic acid)

FIGURE S.1

Selenium is a micromineral that is often considered an antioxidant nutrient. Diets richest in selenium are those of individuals who consume foods from animals that graze in areas with selenium-replete soil. Many regions of China and New Zealand are notorious for having low levels

153

of soil selenium and thus increased risk for selenium deficiency. The roles of selenium in metabolism are centered around its functions with a variety of proteins, often referred to as selenoproteins. Glutathione peroxidase is a key selenoprotein involved in protecting against oxidative damage. Selenium supplementation in athletes has not been extensively studied, but the little available data indicate no effect on exercise performance in rats.[352] The entry for antioxidants describes the relationships among the oxidative stress of exercise, dietary antioxidants, and the body's antioxidant defenses as well as the potential role for supplementation of antioxidant nutrients.

Serine (Figure S.2) is a nonessential amino acid required for the production of the body's proteins. Other functions of serine include the synthesis of ethanolamine and choline, which along with serine and inositol are used to produce various phospholipids. Serine can also be converted to the nonessential amino acid glycine. Potential ergogenic roles of serine have not been identified.

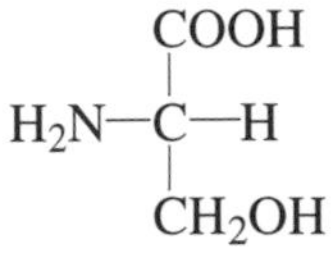

$$COOH$$
$$H_2N-\overset{|}{\underset{|}{C}}-H$$
$$CH_2OH$$

serine

FIGURE S.2

Serotonin (also called 5-hydroxytryptamine) is a neurotransmitter produced in the brain from tryptophan with 5-hydroxytryptophan as an intermediate in the pathway. Serotonin produces changes in mood that can include feelings of sleepiness and mellowness. An increase in serotonin production has been linked to increased uptake of branched chain amino acids by working muscles when carbohydrate stores become depleted. This process has been implicated in the production of fatigue and describes what has been termed the central fatigue theory, which is described more completely in a separate entry.

Short-chain fatty acids Fatty acids with chain lengths of 2 to 4 carbons are considered short-chain fatty acids.

Silicon is a micromineral that is found in whole grains, some vegetables, and beer. It appears to be needed for the development of healthy bones and connective tissue. No studies are available to determine if there is an ergogenic role for silicon.

Simple carbohydrates Carbohydrates with either a single monosaccharide or two monosaccharides linked by a glycosidic bond (disaccharides) are considered simple carbohydrates and are sometimes referred to as simple sugars. Separate entries are provided for the six main simple sugars in the diet, which are glucose, fructose, galactose, sucrose, lactose, and maltose as well as for ribose.

Simple sugars *See* **Simple carbohydrates**

Slow-twitch muscle fiber Muscle fibers that have a slow contractile speed are considered slow-twitch and are also known as type I fibers.

Type I fibers differ from type II fibers, which are considered fast-twitch. Type I fibers, also known as red muscle fibers, primarily produce energy via aerobic metabolism. Type I fibers are often referred to as slow-oxidative (SO) fibers due to their slow contractile speed and their preferred forms of metabolism.

Smilax is considered an anabolic herb due to its sterol content that provides testosterone-like effects according to manufacturers. Anabolic herbs are assumed to be converted in the body into anabolic steroids, and are most commonly used by bodybuilders and weight lifters. However, there is no evidence to support the conversion of plant sterols to testosterone in the human body.[173] In addition, smilax can cause gastric irritation and temporary kidney dysfunction.

Sodium is a macromineral found within the body as the most predominant extracellular cation. In the diet, sodium is typically not present at high levels in fresh foods. Foods with naturally high levels include dairy foods and seafoods, although these are not the richest sources of sodium in the average diet, which provides much higher amounts of sodium from processed foods. Pickles, canned vegetables and soups, soy sauce, preserved meat foods, and many salty snacks are often high in sodium, although low sodium versions of many of these foods are available. Table salt (NaCl) is a particularly rich source, since about 40% of its weight is sodium.

Sodium is essential for electrolyte balance, which controls, at least to some extent, fluid balance, action potentials/nerve transmission, active transport mechanisms, and more. Excess consumption of sodium has been strongly linked to risk for development of hypertension, while low levels of sodium in the blood (hyponatremia) can produce nausea, vomiting, and muscle cramps initially, which can progress to coma and possibly death if not treated. The importance of sodium with regard to replacement of electrolytes during prolonged exercise is discussed in the entry for electrolytes.

Sodium bicarbonate is a chemical compound ($NaHCO_3^-$) used in baking soda and powders and in medicine, especially as an antacid. It is used occasionally by athletes as an ergogenic aid. During near maximal exercise efforts lasting more than 60 seconds, muscles rely on anaerobic metabolism for energy production. Lactic acid is produced in the anaerobic metabolism of glucose, which increases muscular acidity (lowers pH).[352] The accumulation of H^+ in the muscle hinders the release of calcium from the sarcoplasmic reticulum, and reduces the activity of glycolytic enzymes, thereby inhibiting muscular contraction. With the progression of exercise, several buffering mechanisms attempt to counteract this effect, though resulting ultimately in higher

S

amounts of H^+ diffusing into the blood, lowering the pH. Therefore it has been suggested that consumption of bicarbonate in sufficient amounts will increase the buffering capacity and delay fatigue during exercise.[353] It appears that exogenous sodium bicarbonate may assist with transporting lactate and hydrogen ions across the muscle cell membrane during anaerobic exercise, which will result in a smaller decrease in muscle pH, which, as described, tends to have negative effects on muscle performance.[88]

The data in the literature regarding the effects of sodium bicarbonate ingestion before exercise is somewhat conflicted. The inconsistency between different studies has been attributed to differences in the methodologies used, including dosage ingested, time between completion of ingestion and initiation of exercise, exercise protocols, and methodology of controls.[353] Several studies have shown that facilitating a metabolic alkalosis (increased pH) through the ingestion of bicarbonate improves repeated sprint exercise performance and sometimes even an intense single sprint exercise.[354] Other researchers have attempted to demonstrate that bicarbonate can be also effective during prolonged exercise; however, it has been shown that fatigue during prolonged exercise is less likely to be due to acid–base changes but rather has been linked to other effects such as reductions in muscle glycogen availability as well as electrolyte imbalances and dehydration.[354] Nevertheless, some improvements in performance after ingestion of sodium bicarbonate were detected during intermittent exercise performed for a longer duration.[355] Bicarbonate ingestion may therefore improve performance during prolonged intermittent type exercise when pH is repeatedly decreasing to low levels over the course of a long bout of exercise. More research is needed to confirm these results.

The broad conception regarding the effect of sodium bicarbonate ingestion suggests that the most beneficial effects are detected when an adequate dosage is consumed (at least 300 mg per kg body weight) and when the exercise bout is of sufficient duration (between 1 to 7 minutes). In a meta-analysis, 19 studies demonstrated positive effects of ingestion of sodium bicarbonate on performance of primarily anaerobic activities, while 16 studies demonstrated no improvement.[356] Overall, it appears that using sodium bicarbonate as an ergogenic aid in short to medium duration bouts of anaerobic exercise can improve performance by a few seconds under some circumstances. Although these effects seem rather small, they are quite meaningful for athletes for whom even a fraction of a second can be crucial in these types of events.[357]

Although sodium bicarbonate appears to be a beneficial ergogenic aid for some individuals, many athletes find it very difficult if not impossible to compete after ingesting sodium bicarbonate. At least 50% of subjects who participated in studies in which they had to consume sodium bicarbonate reported gastrointestinal distress including vomiting and diarrhea, a fact that should be taken into consideration when weighing the usefulness of sodium bicarbonate as an ergogenic aid.[357]

Sodium citrate The ergogenic potential of sodium citrate has received some attention for its possible effects as a buffer within the body. Consumption of 0.3 to 0.5 g per kg body weight (21 to 35 g in an average 70-kg adult) appears to produce a buffering effect on blood pH.[358] Theoretically, this capacity may have implications for improving performance of activities performed at high intensities for short durations (for example, 400 meter run, 100 to 200 meter swim, etc.). However, much of the available research does not support the use of this substance in enhancing exercise performance,[359–361] while other studies do support the notion of an ergogenic benefit of sodium citrate supplementation.[362–364] It appears that the upper range of the dose required to achieve changes in blood pH balance is most effective in enhancing performance and that the activities most likely improved are short-term, repetitive, exhaustive bouts of exercise.

Spirulina is a blue-green algae that contains protein and various vitamins and minerals. Although spirulina can contribute essential nutrients to the diet, evidence that it can provide an ergogenic effect is lacking.

Sports anemia is a condition that commonly occurs after beginning an exercise program. When initiating such a program, plasma volume typically expands, thereby diluting the concentration of red blood cells and hemoglobin in the blood. In some cases the expansion of plasma volume is sufficient to produces an apparent iron deficiency anemia. Although several studies have actually indicated that exercise training may lead to iron losses through sweat, hemolysis, and gastrointestinal bleeding, in most cases the apparent anemia is simply caused by fluid volume expansion in the blood vessels and is merely transient. Upon adaptation to training, the condition will disappear. For those athletes who have symptoms of anemia well after the initiation of training, consumption of foods rich in iron may be required. Normally menstruating female athletes are of particular concern for true iron deficiency due to monthly losses of iron through menstruation.

Sports bars are often a convenient source of nutrients required by athletes before, during, and after training or competition. Many commercial sports bars are available providing varying amounts of macronutrients and micronutrients. Whether or not a sports bar can provide ergogenic benefits depends upon many factors including their timing of consumption as well as their nutrient content. Entries for carbohydrate and protein provide information that can be used to determine when a sports bar providing carbohydrate and/or protein could be of potential benefit.

Few studies are available to determine if sports bars are truly effective in enhancing performance. One study actually indicated that a commercial bar containing 19 g of carbohydrate, 14 g of protein, and 7 g of fat impaired performance when compared to a feeding providing an equal amount of energy from a glucose polymer.[365]

Sports drinks are typically designed to provide fluid, carbohydrate, and electrolyte replacement. Separate entries are provided for carbohydrate and electrolytes, and the importance of fluids for the prevention of dehydration is described in the entry for hydration. At least 25 commercial sports drinks are available for purchase in the U.S.[366]

An optimal sports drink will promote consumption of fluid and nutrients through palatability and will provide appropriate ingredients to meet the athletes' needs (for example, hydration, energy, electrolytes, etc.) for a particular event with no ingredients included that can limit intake or performance or unnecessarily add to the cost of the beverage. The formulation of the sports drink will impact each of these factors.

To maximize hydration, a fluid should be palatable, thus promoting its consumption. Research suggests that a beverage that is sweetened, flavored, and provides some sodium may most enhance consumption. The fluid should also maximize water absorption. Fluids too high in osmolality (concentration of solute particles in a solution) can produce a lower rate of water absorption; thus, fluids should be isotonic or hypotonic, depending on the other characteristics required of the sports drink. Some evidence suggests that including sodium in a sports drink may enhance intake by providing a physiological thirst response due to increased vascular sodium concentration.[367] One factor that may limit hydration by decreasing intake is carbonation, which may produce a sense of fullness; however, light carbonation does not appear to decrease fluid intake and can contribute to palatability for some individuals.[368]

During training or events in which an important function of the sports drink is to provide energy (usually those lasting about 1 hour or longer), the formulation should provide an optimal amount of readily available energy with least risk of malabsorption. Carbohydrate is typically considered the optimal macronutrient to provide energy in a sports drink. Solutions with lower concentrations of carbohydrate are typically best absorbed. When the concentration of carbohydrate surpasses 6 to 7%, water absorption can be limited and gastrointestinal distress can occur. Some research has suggested that carbohydrates in the form of glucose polymers may provide a benefit for fluid absorption due to providing a lower osmalality of the solution.[292] Other studies indicate that glucose, sucrose, glucose polymers (maltodextrins), or combinations of these carbohydrates with or without fructose provide relatively equal ergogenic benefits. When fructose is fed alone, it may promote gastrointestinal distress since it is absorbed by a saturable facilitated diffusion process; thus, it is recommended only when in combination with other carbohydrates. Furthermore, combinations of various carbohydrate sources appear to promote absorption of fluids and enhance the rate of monosaccharide availability and utilization.[369]

Electrolyte content (sodium, potassium, and chloride in particular) can be an important consideration for sports drinks. Popular commercial sports drinks typically provide 55 to 110 mg of sodium and 30 to 55 mg of potassium per 8 oz. Although for some athletes the concentrations of these electrolytes in the sweat may exceed the concentration in these beverages, reports of hyponatremia or hypokalemia in athletes using commercial sports drinks to meet 100% of sweat losses are extremely rare. In most cases, loss of electrolytes does not typically pose a problem during competition or training unless the exercise is of a prolonged nature or in conditions of high ambient temperatures or humidity. However, as stated earlier, sodium may also be beneficial within a sports drink by virtue of its tendency to promote thirst and fluid intake. Excess sodium on the other hand appears to limit fluid intake either by promoting increased vascular volume or by decreasing fluid palatability.[370]

Some commercial sports drinks provide other ingredients that may or may not impact performance. Some additional ingredients include vitamins, amino acids, glycerol, caffeine, and herbals. Separate entries regarding the potential ergogenic benefits of many of these ingredients are provided throughout this book.

Sports gels are carbohydrate-rich semisolids used to replenish glucose utilized during exercise. Some sports gels contain vitamins, amino acids, glycerol, caffeine, herbals, and other constituents, also. Separate entries regarding the potential ergogenic benefits of many of these ingredients are provided throughout this book.

Commercial sports gels vary in their total contents and types of carbohydrates. These differences can elicit varying physiological responses, since many of the carbohydrates used vary in glycemic index. Sports gels likely provide no advantage, other than convenience in some cases, over many whole foods.

Sports nutrition encompasses all aspects of the study of nutrition for athletes. This includes but is not limited to assessment of dietary intake and nutritional status of athletes, determination of dietary principles, nutrients and supplements that impact exercise performance, and counseling athletes for optimal dietary intake.

Proper nutrition is vital for optimal athletic performance. Clinical deficiency of any nutrient and subclinical deficiency of most are likely to impair performance. Conversely, nutritional excesses that lead to toxic effects or overweight/obesity will likely impair performance as well. Although the nutrient needs of active vs. inactive individuals has not been well-studied for most nutrients, the keys to proper nutrition for athletes are very similar to those of nonathletes. The entry on dietary recommendations for athletes provides an overview of general nutritional guidelines.

Starch Starches are long, sometimes highly branched-chains of glucose units (polysaccharides) linked by glycosidic bonds. Amylose and amylopectin are polyscaccharides that are collectively referred to as starches. Figures S.3 and S.4 depict the structures of amylose and amylopectin, respectively.

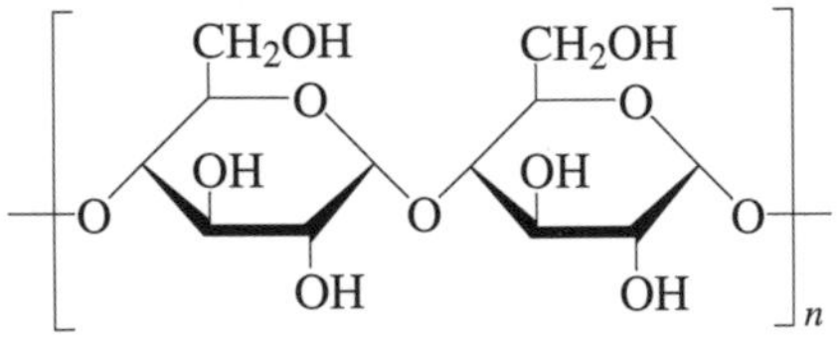

amylose

FIGURE S.3

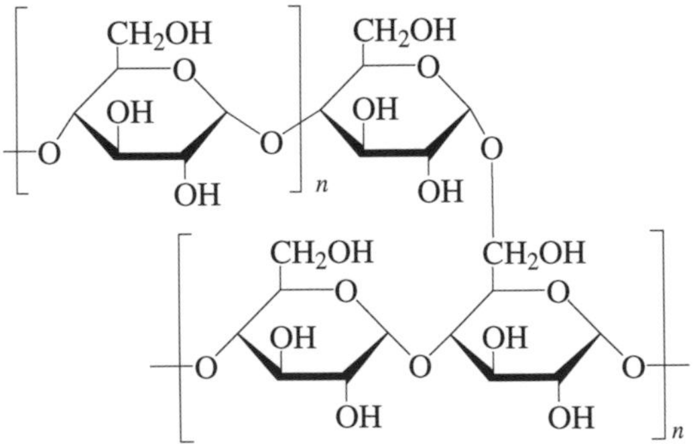

S

amylopectin

FIGURE S.4

Steroids Anabolic steroid drugs are hormones and hormonal precursors that produce elevations in or mimic the functions of testosterone. They are often used illegally to produce increases in weight, lean body mass, and strength. Since steroids are oral or injectable pharmacological and not nutritional agents, detailed descriptions of the research regarding steroids is beyond the scope of this book. In general, however, steroids are androgenic compounds capable of increasing weight and when used during resistance training can lead to increased lean body mass. Many studies support the potential for steroids to increase strength as well. Negative effects of anabolic-androgenic steroids include alterations to liver function, increased risk of cardiovascular disease, altered reproduction and reproductive organs, development of acne, and mental instability. Overall, since steroids are illegal by law and for competition and can produce many negative side effects, the positive influence on strength gains and increases in lean body mass are far outweighed.

Substrate A substrate is a substance that is required for and participates in a biochemical reaction.

Sucrose (Figure S.5) is a disaccharide produced from one unit of glucose and one unit of fructose. It is found in high levels in sugar cane and sugar beets from which it is processed to produce table sugar. It is also found in lower amounts in many fruits as well as vegetables and grains. Sucrose is digested to its complementary monosaccharides primarily by the enzyme sucrase, which is secreted at the brush border of the small intestine.

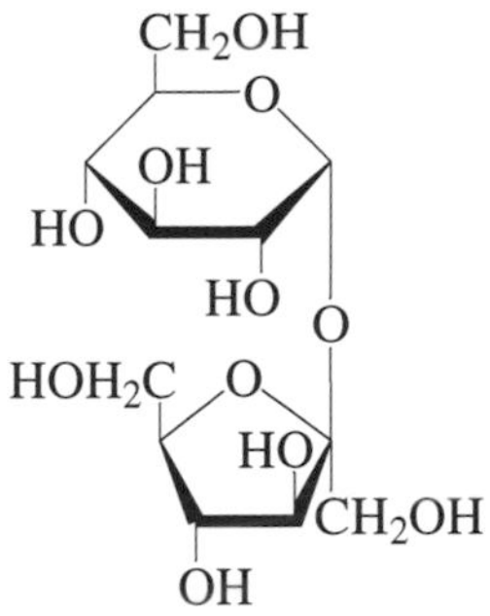

sucrose

FIGURE S.5

Sugar The term sugar is often used in a variety of ways. Sometimes it is used to describe carbohydrates in general, while other times it is used to describe a particular simple carbohydrate, such as glucose when discussing blood sugar. Most often sugar is used to refer to table sugar, which is the disaccharide sucrose.

Sulfur is a macromineral found in highest concentrations in protein-rich foods including meat, fish, poultry, eggs, dairy foods, legumes, and nuts. A primary role of sulfur is serving as a structural component of important compounds including the sulfur-containing amino acids, thiamin, biotin, lipoic acid, and some proteins integral in metabolism. Sulfur is also involved in energy production as part of iron–sulfur complexes found in the electron transport chain.

Supplements *See* **Dietary supplements**

Synephrine is considered a biogenic amine that appears to have metabolic effects similar to epinephrine. It is commonly obtained by ingestion of citrus arantium, an herb marketed as a fat loss aid. Little research is available regarding the influence of oral synephrine supplementation and there are no studies available that assess its potential to enhance athletic performance.

Sweat is the fluid produced in and secreted from the sweat glands of the skin. Sweat is primarily water, but is a serous fluid containing many of the same constituents as plasma. Most importantly with respect to sports nutrition, sweat contains relatively high concentrations of electrolytes. During periods of excess sweating, fluid and electrolytes may be depleted to a great extent, requiring their replacement through the diet. Entries for hydration and electrolytes as well as sports drinks provide some detail regarding effective fluid and electrolyte replacement.

S

T

Taurine is a sulfur-containing nonessential amino acid synthesized from methionine. Unlike most amino acids, it is not incorporated into the proteins of the body. Taurine is available from the diet and is found in relatively high concentrations in intracellular fluids. Taurine is involved in conjugation of bile acids; however, other potential functions including central nervous system neuromodulation, retinal development and function, endocrine effects, and antioxidant properties are less clearly understood. A role for taurine supplementation for exercise performance has not been established; however, one study in which taurine (0.5 g/kg body weight) was added to the water of rats for 2 weeks suggested that supplementation may improve treadmill running to exhaustion perhaps by maintaining muscle concentration of taurine,[371] which has been demonstrated to be decreased by exercise.[372]

Testosterone is an androgenic steroid hormone ultimately synthesized from cholesterol. It is especially important for male reproduction and development of typical male characteristics.

Thiamin (Figure T.1), also known as vitamin B_1, is a water-soluble vitamin that is extremely important for obtaining energy from macronutrients, particularly carbohydrate. It carries out much of its functions within the body in a phosphorylated form called thiamin diphosphate (TDP), which is required for function of the pyruvate dehydrogenase complex and Krebs cycle. Thiamin is also required for function of the enzyme transketolase, which assists in the production of ribose from glucose through the hexosemonophosphate shunt.

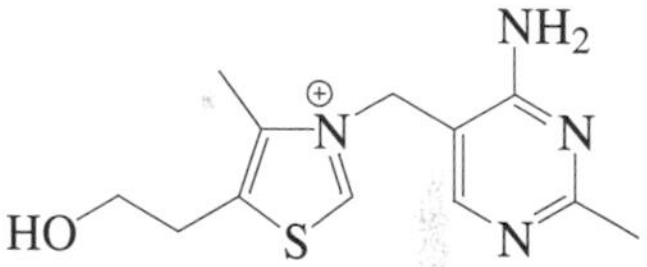

thiamine (vitamin B_1)

FIGURE T.1

Since thiamin, like many B-vitamins, is needed for obtaining energy from food, it has been targeted as an ergogenic aid. Although it is unlikely that thiamin supplementation affects exercise performance,[314,373] one study that administered extremely high doses of thiamin (900 mg/day) suggests that thiamin may alter metabolic processes related to performance.[374] Some changes included increased anaerobic threshold, decreased accumulation of blood lactic acid, and reduced heart rate during exercise. These effects have not been demonstrated consistently and no studies indicate that thiamin actually improves exercise performance.

Threonine (Figure T.2) is an essential amino acid containing a hydroxyl group. Threonine is required for the formation of the body's proteins. Potential ergogenic roles of threonine supplementation have not been identified.

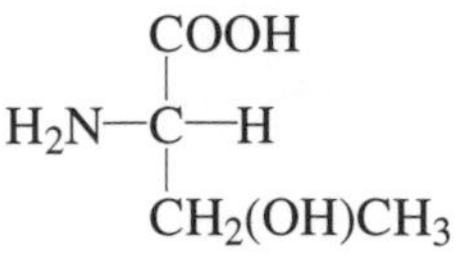

$$COOH$$
$$H_2N-C-H$$
$$CH_2(OH)CH_3$$

threonine

FIGURE T.2

Tocopherol *See* **Vitamin E**

Tolerable Upper Intake Level (UL) The Tolerable Upper Intake Level is one of four possible Dietary Reference Intake (DRI) values established by the Food and Nutrition Board of the National Academy of Sciences. The UL is the highest level of daily intake for a nutrient that is likely to cause no adverse health effects in almost all individuals within a particular age range. Consumption of nutrients at levels of intake above the UL is not recommended.

Trace minerals are microminerals required in minute amounts in the diet.

Trans **fatty acids** are more accurately called *trans* unsaturated fatty acids, since they possess at least one double bond in unsaturated fatty acids. The hydrogen molecules on the double-bonded carbons can be oriented either on the same side of the hydrocarbon chain or on the opposite side. Fatty acids with a *trans* configuration have hydrogen atoms oriented across from one another, which produces a hydrocarbon that takes on what is considered a straight structure, unlike those with a *cis* configuration that possess what has been called a bend in the hydrocarbon chain. These differences in structure produce vastly different effects on metabolism, with most *trans* unsaturated fatty acids producing harmful effects relative to *cis* unsaturated fatty acids.

Trehalose is a disaccharide composed of two glucose molecules bound via the number 1 carbon of the two glucose units. Trehalose is not found in high quantities in the diet but has been detected in foods such as mushrooms, honey, shrimp, lobster, and foods made with yeasts. One study has determined that feeding trehalose 45 minutes prior to cycling exercise produces a lower glycemic and insulinemic response in comparison to glucose.[375] However, no difference in cycling performance was detected in that study.

Tribulus terrestris is marketed for unproven testosterone-enhancing capabilities. Very little research is available regarding its ergogenic potential; however, one study in which resistance-trained men consumed an herbal preparation containing 3.21 mg of *Tribulus* per kg of body weight failed to demonstrate enhancements in body weight and composition, strength, or mood states.[376] In fact, the placebo group outperformed the *Tribulus* group following supplementation in one measure of strength.

Triglycerides (also known as triacylglycerols) consist of a 3-carbon glycerol backbone bound to three fatty acids. Triglycerides account for the vast majority of dietary lipids and provide energy as well as essential fatty acids to the body.

Tripeptide A tripeptide is three amino acids linked together by peptide bonds.

Tryptophan (Figure T.3) is an essential aromatic amino acid needed for synthesis of the body's proteins. It also serves other important roles in metabolism, including the synthesis of niacin as well as serotonin. Tryptophan and its metabolite 5-hydroxytryptophan have been marketed for their ergogenic potential due to their roles in serotonin production.

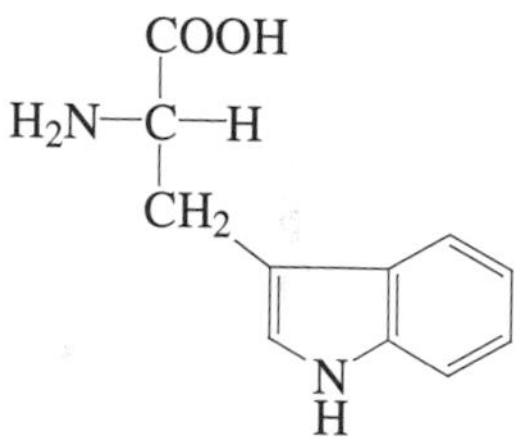

$$H_2N-\underset{\underset{CH_2}{|}}{\overset{\overset{COOH}{|}}{C}}-H$$

tryptophan

FIGURE T.3

Serotonin (also called 5-hydroxytryptamine) is a neurotransmitter produced in the brain. It is best known for producing changes in mood that can include feelings of sleepiness and a calming effect. Some individuals have speculated that this altered mood state may decrease pain perception and allow an athlete to work harder without succumbing to the pain of strenuous activity. One study in which 1.2 g of tryptophan were fed over a period of 24 hours reported a lower rating of perceived exertion during strenuous activity, as well as an improvement in endurance.[377] The authors detected a 49% improvement in performance, however, which has been criticized since that is well beyond any improvement that could have been predicted. Subsequent research detected no differences in performance between tryptophan intake at the same level and a placebo[378] as well as when performance was assessed with tryptophan added to sucrose vs. sucrose alone.[86] Another study suggested that opposite results with regard to perceived fatigue occurred with consumption of 30 mg tryptophan per kg body weight vs. a placebo.[379] Interestingly, grip strength was greater following tryptophan consumption, which the researchers speculated may have been due to decreased levels of discomfort.

T

As described in the entry for the central fatigue theory, an increase in serotonin production from tryptophan has been linked to increased uptake of branched-chain amino acids by working muscles when carbohydrate stores are depleted. This process has been implicated in the production of fatigue. If correct, this theory would suggest that tryptophan supplementation is more likely to be ergolytic than ergogenic.

Tyrosine (Figure T.4) is an essential amino acid containing a hydroxyl group. Tyrosine is required for the formation of the body's proteins and can be metabolized to a variety of neurotransimitters and hormones including L-DOPA, dopamine, norepinephrine, epinephrine, melanin, and thyroid hormone.

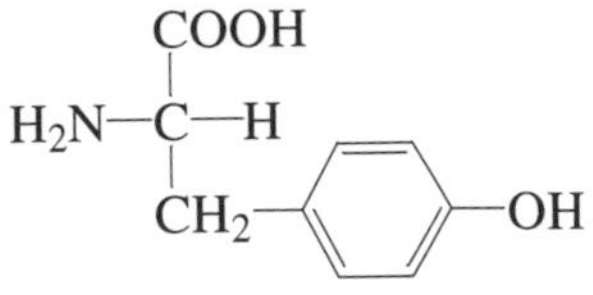

tyrosine

FIGURE T.4

Potential ergogenic roles of tyrosine supplementation have not been well-researched. In one study tyrosine supplementation was compared to branched-chain amino acid supplementation with regard to potential to influence endurance performance.[380] Twenty grams of tyrosine were fed prior to exercise in that study and compared to a separate occasion in which 21 g of a mixture of branched-chain amino acids were fed. Both trials were also compared to a placebo trial as well as a trial in which paroxetine (a serotonin reuptake inhibitor) was given. No differences in exercise performance were detected among the placebo, tyrosine, and branched-chain amino acid trials, although endurance was greater in each of these trials compared to the paroxetine trial.

In another study, 75 mg of tyrosine per kg body weight were supplemented over a 1-hour period in a solution with or without glucose polymers prior to 90 minutes of exercise.[381] This was followed by a time trial for performance. When carbohydrate was fed either with or without tyrosine, endurance was enhanced compared to tyrosine feeding alone and a placebo trial.

The research to date suggests that although tyrosine is a vital precursor to hormones that are integral for metabolism, such as epinephrine, even massive doses are insufficient to elicit an enhancement in exercise performance. At this time there appears to be no ergogenic role for tyrosine supplementation.

U

Ubiquinone *See* **Coenzyme Q**
UL *See* **Tolerable Upper Intake Level**
Unsaturated fatty acids Fatty acids are commonly classified based on their degree of saturation with hydrogen atoms, which is determined by the absence or presence of double bonds between carbon atoms. Unsaturated fatty acids have at least one double bond in their chain, which prevents saturation of the hydrocarbon chain hydrogen ions. Monounsaturated fatty acids have a single double bond, while polyunsaturated fatty acids have two or more double bonds.

V

Valine (Figure V.1) is a branched-chain, essential amino acid. It is needed for synthesis of proteins and can be used for energy production within the muscle cell as well. Metabolism of valine in the muscle results in the eventual production of propionyl CoA, which can be converted to succinyl CoA (an intermediate of Krebs cycle).

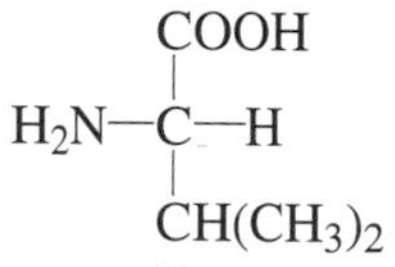

$$
\begin{array}{c}
COOH \\
| \\
H_2N-C-H \\
| \\
CH(CH_3)_2
\end{array}
$$

valine

FIGURE V.1

Since catabolism of branched-chain amino acids may be important in producing central fatigue, as described in a separate entry, many studies have examined their ergogenic potential. While some researchers have provided individual branched-chain amino acids to their participants, most have fed the compounds as mixtures. Research on the potential ergogenic benefits of their supplementation is described in the entry for branched-chain amino acids.

Vanadium is a micromineral found in trace amounts within the body and the diet. Food sources most rich in vanadium include spinach, shellfish, black pepper, mushrooms, and parsley. Vanadium has not been established as an essential nutrient; however, it has been demonstrated to have functions similar to those of insulin in humans with non-insulin-dependent diabetes mellitus. Those effects include decreased blood glucose concentrations during fasting, increased insulin-mediated glucose uptake, and increased muscle glycogen synthesis. Since insulin is an important anabolic hormone and vanadium may produce similar effects in diabetic subjects, vanadium, particularly as vanadyl sulfate, has been marketed for its potential to increase lean body mass and strength in athletes as well as optimize glycogen stores.

Although there are several studies showing some insulin-like benefits of vanadium supplements in humans with diabetes, similar results do not occur in healthy humans[382]; thus, an ergogenic benefit for nondiabetic individuals would be unlikely. Research that has directly assessed potential ergogenic effects has detected no effects of 12 weeks of vanadium supplementation at 0.5 mg/kg body weight on body composition.[383] Measures of strength were also performed and vanadium produced little if any effect. In one of four strength tests, a significant increase in the vanadium-supplemented group was detected; however, the authors discredited this result since it appeared that the group underperformed in the baseline test performed prior to vanadium supplementation, whereas it performed equally to the placebo group at baseline for all other measures of strength. No differences in strength between the vanadium and placebo-supplemented groups were detected after supplementation for any of the four measures.

Vanadyl sulfate *See* **Vanadium**

Vegan A vegan is a vegetarian who avoids all animal foods including meats, fish, poultry, eggs, and dairy foods.

Vegetarian A vegetarian is an individual whose diet is based solely or primarily on plant foods. Several levels of vegetarianism exist, but the most typical are vegans, lactovegeterians, ovovegetarians, and lactoovovegeterians. A vegan is a vegetarian who avoids all animal foods including meats, fish, poultry, eggs, and dairy foods. A lactovegetarian will consume dairy foods in addition to plant foods, but will not consume meats, fish, poultry, or eggs. An ovovegetarian will consume eggs in addition to plant foods, but will not consume meats, fish, poultry, or dairy foods. A lactoovovegetarian will consume both dairy foods and eggs in addition to plant foods.

All of the above types of vegetarians can consume a diet adequate to meet their needs for normal growth, development, and athletic performance. Vegans must be particularly mindful of their food selection, however, since few foods other than dairy products provide

U–V

vitamin D and unless fortified, only animal foods will provide vitamin B_{12}. These nutrients should be obtained by a selection of fortified foods and or supplementation, although much of the vitamin D requirements can be met through exposure of the skin to sunlight.

Vinpocetine is a synthetic ethyl ester of apovincamine and is among the family of drugs called vinco alkaloids. It has been used to improve cerebral perfusion of acute stroke survivors; however, it is not clear if it is an effective treatment.[384]

Research regarding the ergogenic potential of vinpocetine or other vincamines is unavailable. Vinpocetine appears to have alpha 2- and alpha 1-adrenoceptor blocking actions and increases norepinephrine when injected.[385] Oral supplementation has not been demonstrated to produce similar effects or enhance exercise performance.

Vitamin A (Figure V.2) is a fat-soluble vitamin that is best known as a requirement for normal vision. It is also needed for other functions including cell differentiation and function, immune responses, and reproduction. Carotenoids, dark orange pigments, can be used to produce the vitamin, but are also potent antioxidants. A separate entry is provided for beta-carotene, which is a major carotenoid in the diet that produces vitamin A more efficiently than other carotenoids. Vitamin A is found in many animal products and is especially rich in eggs and fortified dairy foods. Carotenoids tend to be found at high levels in dark orange and dark green fruits and vegetables. Deficiency of vitamin A can produce night-blindness and many other clinical symptoms. Although a deficient state is likely to impair performance, supplementation does not appear to enhance endurance.[386] The antioxidant properties of beta-carotene have been an area of interest for preventing oxidative stress in exercisers. The entry for antioxidants provides a description of potential roles of beta-carotene supplementation for athletes.

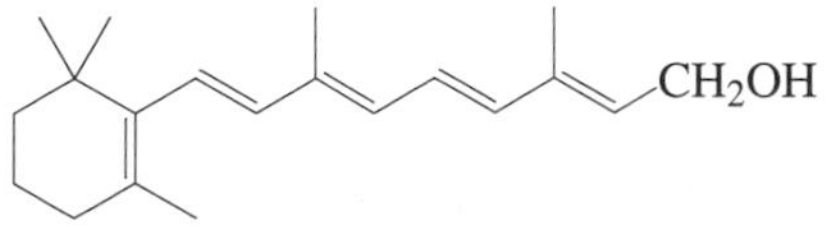

CH₂OH

vitamin A

FIGURE V.2

U–V

Vitamin B$_1$ *See* **Thiamin**
Vitamin B$_2$ *See* **Riboflavin**
Vitamin B$_3$ *See* **Niacin**
Vitamin B$_5$ *See* **Pantothenic acid**
Vitamin B$_6$ (Figure V.3) is actually a term used to describe a group of three water-soluble vitamers (pyridoxine, pyridoxal, and pyridoxamine), each of which can also be found in their phosphorylated forms. Vitamin B$_6$ is particularly important as a cofactor for enzymatic reactions. Functions of this vitamin include amino acid metabolism, heme formation, glyco-

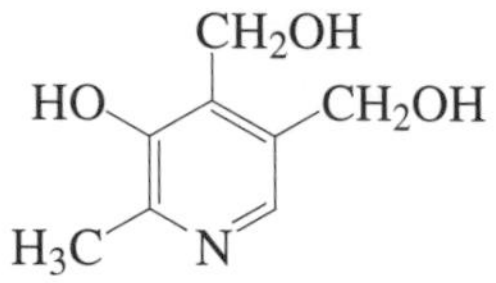

pyridoxine (vitamin B$_6$)

FIGURE V.3

genolysis, niacin synthesis, and more. Deficiency can produce many symptoms incuding fatigue, due to hypochromic, microcytic anemia from the decreased capability to synthesize heme. Dietary sources of vitamin B$_6$ include meat, fish, poultry, beans, potatoes, and bananas.

    When supplemented at 8 to 10 g/day along with a high carbohydrate diet, vitamin B$_6$ may improve glycogen utilization and lower free fatty acid concentrations.[387] While some claim that this effect could be potentially ergogenic, it is more likely to decrease endurance exercise performance and thus be classified as an ergolytic substance. Therefore, supplementation of large doses is not recommended. Additionally, since excess B$_6$ can cause liver disease and nerve damage, megadoses are not recommended.[388]

Vitamin B$_{12}$ (see Figure V.4) is a group of water-soluble molecules called cobalamins, which get their name from the mineral cobalt. Cobalt is the central atom of the vitamin's structure. Vitamin B$_{12}$ is particularly important for DNA synthesis and cell division. Dietary deficiency produces a megaloblastic anemia, which can also be caused by low production of instrinsic factor, a protein synthesized in the stomach that is needed for absorption of B$_{12}$ in the small intestine. When this occurs, the deficiency syndrome is referred to as pernicious anemia. Either form of deficiency can result in decreased exercise performance due to poor oxygen delivery to the tissues. Dietary B$_{12}$ is limited to animal foods and foods that are fortified with the vitamin. Supplements of B$_{12}$ have been marketed for their ergogenic potential for years; however, research has not demonstrated that B$_{12}$ can improve performance even as injections of cyanocobalamin.[389]

U–V

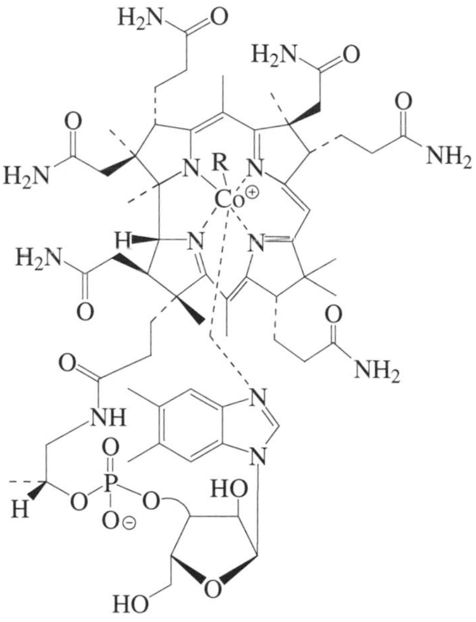

vitamin B$_{12}$

FIGURE V.4

R = CN

Vitamin C (Figure V.5), also referred to as ascorbic acid, is a water-soluble vitamin that acts as an antioxidant in the body and performs various other functions as a cofactor for enzymes. Biochemical processes that require vitamin C include collagen synthesis, carnitine production, and tyrosine metabolism in the synthesis of neurotransmitters and hormones. Deficiency can produce fatigue and muscular weakness and ultimately scurvy, which is characterized by bleeding gums and impaired wound healing. Dietary vitamin C is primarily provided in fruits and vegetables including citrus fruits, peppers, broccoli, potatoes, tomatoes, and others.

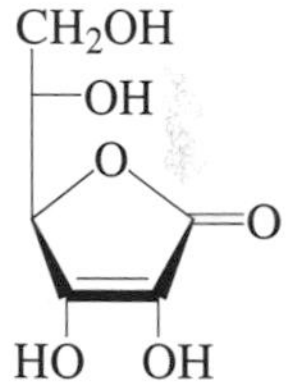

ascorbic acid (vitamin C)

FIGURE V.5

The antioxidative potential of vitamin C has been theorized to protect muscles from oxidative damage that may occur during exercise. The entry for antioxidants provides more information for the potential importance of antioxidants for exercisers and athletes.

Several studies assessing the potential ergogenic characteristics of vitamin C have been conducted as summarized by Bucci.[390] In general, most of these studies reported no effects in either performance or performance-related physiology. Of the remaining studies summarized, six detected some potential benefits including increased strength, increased submaximal work efficiency, decreased energy expenditure, ventilation and heart rate, increased work capacity, and decreased blood lactate concentrations. Negative effects were reported in three studies including decreased aerobic capacity and decreased strength. Neither dosage nor duration of administration seemed to determine the outcomes of the study. Bucci concludes that many of the studies were experimentally flawed and that better designed research is needed to obtain a conclusive decision regarding the potential benefits of vitamin C supplementation and the level and duration required if an ergogenic effect is possible.

Vitamin D The active form of vitamin D, a fat-soluble vitamin synthesized from cholesterol, is known as calcitriol or 1,25-dihydroxycholecalciferol (Figure V.6). Vitamin D is important for cell differentiation and immune function but is primarily known for its roles in calcium metabolism. These roles include enhancing calcium absorption at the small intestine, increasing calcium retention by the kidney, and elevating calcium mobilization

vitamin D_3

FIGURE V.6

from the bone. Vitamin D deficiency is linked to bone demineralization, which can produce rickets in children and osteomalacia and possibly osteoporosis in adults. Much of our requirement for vitamin D can be acquired by exposure of the skin to sunlight, which allows for production of an inactive form of vitamin D from cholesterol that can be metabolized by the liver and then kidney to the active form. Vitamin D is found in some fatty animal foods, but the majority of dietary vitamin D is obtained from fortified dairy foods. There are no known mechanisms by which vitamin D supplementation may enhance performance of athletes. Furthermore, vitamin D is considered quite toxic at high doses.

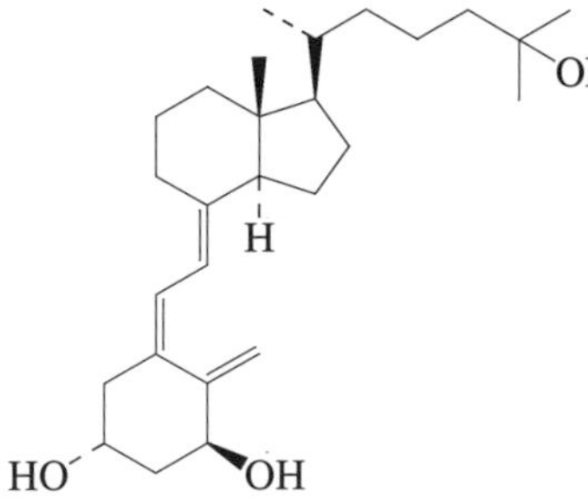

Vitamin E Several forms of vitamin E (see Figure V.7) varying in activity have been identified including the alpha, beta, gamma, and delta forms of tocopherols and tocotrienols, which are fat-soluble. Alpha-tocopherol

U–V

is generally considered the most active form. Vitamin E is a powerful antioxidant and is particularly protective against lipid oxidation. Since the antioxidant properties of vitamin E can prevent destruction of lipid-rich cellular membranes, deficiency can produce hemolytic anemia in which red blood cells become fragile and are susceptible to breaking. This can result in diminished physical work capacity.

Common dietary sources of vitamin E include vegetable oils, particularly those rich in polyunsaturated fatty acids, nuts, seeds, whole grains, and green, leafy vegetables. Studies in swimmers do not support vitamin E as a supplement capable of improving exercise performance.[31-35] However, some research suggests that blood lactate concentrations may be lowered by supplementation, which may have implications for performance.[391] The majority of research regarding vitamin E supplementation for athletes revolves around its antioxidant potential. The roles of vitamin E as an antioxidant for athletes are described in the entry for antioxidants.

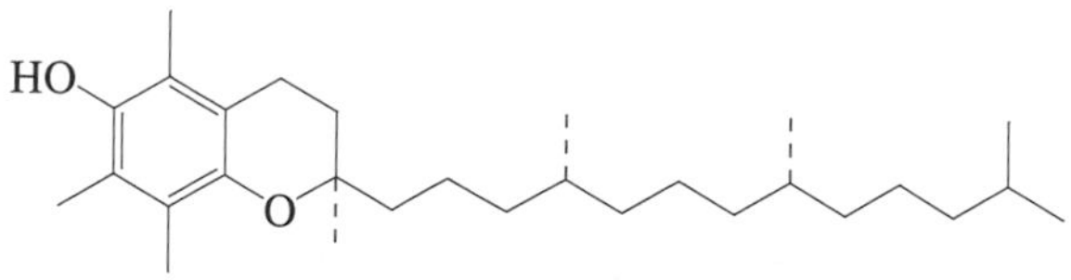

vitamin E

FIGURE V.7

Vitamin K (Figure V.8), also referrred to as phylloquinone as the naturally occuring form in plants, is a fat-soluble vitamin needed for normal blood clotting and bone formation. Deficiency is linked to increased risk of hemorrhage as well as osteoporosis. Most dietary vitamin K is obtained from leafy, green vegetables such as spinach, lettuce and other salad greens, kale, collard greens, and broccoli, as well as other vegetables and legumes. Potential ergogenic roles of vitamin K have not been identified.

U–V

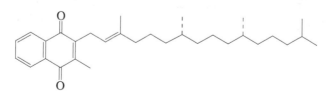

vitamin K

FIGURE V.8

Vitamins are organic molecules that are required in the diet but only in minute amounts. Although some vitamins can be synthesized by the human body (such as niacin from tryptophan, vitamin D from cholesterol, vitamin A from carotenoids, and perhaps choline from serine and methionine) or by bacteria within the colon (such as vitamin K, biotin, etc.), the amount produced is usually inadequate to meet the full demands of the body. Although many vitamins as well as multivitamins have been marketed as ergogenic aids, well-designed studies have largely failed to support the need for supplementation of any vitamin in nondeficient athletes. For each vitamin, it is very likely that a clinical deficiency will impair athletic performance in some way.

It is possible that under certain circumstances and with the correct dose and timing of intake that some vitamins could someday prove to be ergogenic. However, with today's state of science it appears that adequate vitamin intake to prevent a deficiency is all that is required. See entries for each vitamin for further information regarding potential influences of exercise on vitamin status and on vitamin supplementation and performance.

Vitamin toxicity Excess consumption of some vitamins can produce toxic effects. Vitamins A and D are typically considered the most potentially toxic. Daily vitamin intake should not exceed the Tolerable Upper Intake Level (UL) established by the Food and Nutrition Board of the National Academy of Sciences for those vitamins for which a UL has been set.

$VO_{2\,max}$ *See* **Maximal oxygen consumption**

W

Water *See* **Hydration status**

Water-soluble vitamins Vitamins that dissolve in aqueous solvents are considered water-soluble vitamins and include ascorbic acid, thiamin, riboflavin, niacin, vitamin B_6, vitamin B_{12}, folic acid, pantothenic acid, and biotin. In general water-soluble vitamins are absorbed through the portal blood supply. Within the bloodstream, water-soluble vitamins are often transported unbound although many are also present in the blood as their coenzyme forms or bound to transport proteins. Clinical deficiency of any of the water-soluble vitamins is likely to impair athletic performance; however, research supporting a benefit for their supplementation to improve performance is scant at best.

Weight-conscious athletes Many athletes seek to lose weight or maintain a low body weight for competition. For example, wrestlers, boxers, rowers, jockeys, and other athletes often compete in events in which there are rigorous weight requirements or specified weight classes that can not be exceeded for participation. Other athletes, such as gymnasts, ballet dancers, and bodybuilders, participate in sports in which they are judged on aesthetics in movement and form. Many of these athletes are often preoccupied by their body weight, are more likely to have nutritional inadequacies, and appear to be more predisposed to disordered eating (such as anorexia nervosa and bulimia nervosa).[392]

Basic dietary recommendations for weight-conscious athletes are typically not different from those of other athletes. Diets based on the Food Guide Pyramid can provide all of the nutrients needed to allow the athlete to perform optimally. These athletes are less likely than other athletes to consume appropriate diets. To maximize performance, practitioners should pay particularly close attention to the dietary habits of these athletes. Additionally, the practitioner should be aware of warning signs that can indicate that the athlete is suffering from an eating disorder. Although disordered eating is more prevalent in weight-conscious athletes, the practitioner should keep in mind that eating disorders also occur in other types of athletes as well.

Eating disorders are extremely complex problems. Symptoms vary among eating disorder types but often include: 1) low body weight; 2) being overly concerned about body weight or having a fear of fatness; 3) having a distorted body image; 4) having abnormal eating habits that may include restrained eating, binge eating, or purging; 5) preoccupation with food; and 6) abnormal or loss of menstruation. Disordered eating can devastate athletic performance, but effects on health can be much more severe. Practitioners should be knowledgeable of the local resources available to athletes who have disordered eating tendencies. Treatment of individuals diagnosed with an eating disorder usually requires a team approach including the services of a physician, psychologist, registered dietitian, and possibly other health-care workers. More information regarding disordered eating and its effects is available in the entries for eating disorders and the female athlete triad.

Weight gain occurs when energy intake exceeds energy expenditure. Many factors can affect either energy intake or expenditure and produce increased body weight. Some athletes desire weight gain for improved performance, while others prefer to avoid weight gain. Most often, athletes wishing to gain weight are interested in adding lean body mass. Other athletes, such as sumo wrestlers or perhaps football linemen, may simply wish to add extra pounds and may or may not require increased lean body mass concurrently to achieve their goals.

Weight gain in general is rather simple to achieve, but when the goal is to add lean body mass, the task is more difficult. As with any weight gain, in order to gain weight as lean body mass, energy intake must exceed energy expenditure. For gains in lean tissue, energy intake must meet at least three added energy demands. One is the increased energy expenditure of resistance training, which is required for muscle cell hypertrophy and possibly hyperplasia. Another is the energy content of the additional tissue itself. The third is the energy for biochemical reactions that produce the tissue.

Considering these three factors and many variables that will affect the production of lean tissue, the actual amount of energy that is required to produce an given amount of lean body mass is unclear. However, an additional 2500 to 3500 kcal above energy expenditure (taking into consideration energy expenditure of the resistance training) over a period of time of at least 1 week is typically considered sufficient to add an additional pound of lean weight. The rate of weight gain will be determined in large part by genetic potential and the volume of resistance training performed.

Weight loss occurs when energy expenditure exceeds energy intake. Many factors can affect either energy intake or energy expenditure and lead to loss of body weight. A comprehensive review of factors involved in weight loss is beyond the scope of this book; however, some general principals, particularly related to athletes, will be provided.

Athletes may desire weight loss for a variety of reasons. In some cases the athlete must meet a specific weight maximum to compete within a particular weight class. Others desire weight loss for asthetic purposes, to increase mechanical efficiency, for health, or for many other reasons. Athletes who are chronically concerned about body weight should be treated differently than athletes who attempt to lose weight on an infrequent basis. These weight-conscious athletes are discussed in a separate entry under that name.

Weight loss can be achieved by either decreasing energy intake or increasing energy expenditure. In athletes who are already training heavily, weight loss is most likely to be safely accomplished by a mild to moderate energy restriction rather than an increase in energy expenditure within an already strenuous training program. The goal of weight loss for athletes is to maximize fat loss while minimizing loss of lean tissue. While preserving 100% of lean tissue is difficult during weight loss, the slower the rate of weight loss, the better the chances that lean tissue will be preserved. In average individuals, a recommended range for safe weight loss is typically 1 to 2 lb per week.[393]

One pound of weight loss typically occurs with an energy deficit of approximately 3500 kcal. Although 1 lb of pure fat (triglyceride) is equal to approximately 4086 kcal, this value should not be used to determine pounds of weight loss since 100% of weight loss is not from fat. To achieve a 3500 kcal energy deficit, a) caloric intake can be restricted to a level that would result in a deficit over a few days; b) energy expenditure could be increased by increasing physical activity; or c) a combination of both could be used.

When possible, weight loss should be planned while the athlete is not involved in the competitive season for two major reasons. One reason is that weight loss out of the season may provide the athlete with ample time to rebuild any lost lean tissue. Another is that energy restriction could compromise energy stores, which could produce inferior performances if weight is lost during the season.

Wheat germ oil The wheat germ is the portion of the wheat grain that contains the embryo and relatively high fat content. Wheat germ oil is extracted from the wheat germ and is available as a dietary supplement. Well-designed research does not support an ergogenic effect of wheat germ oil. Octacosanol, a 28-carbon alcohol in wheat germ oil, is often cited as the active ingredient and is described in a separate entry.

Whey protein is obtained from milk and is commonly marketed to enhance lean body mass of athletes who include resistance training in their workouts. As described in the entry for proteins, there is little research avaible to suggest that bodybuilders can synthesize more muscle from one protein than another. On the other hand, two studies have reported that casein may be used preferentially for body protein synthesis when compared to whey.[334,335] In that research, the two proteins were fed to resting participants on separate occasions following an overnight fasting. Over a period of several hours, blood and breath collections revealed that whey protein was digested and absorbed more rapidly and was more likely to be metabolized for energy than casein and that casein was more likely to be used for protein synthesis. These studies did not demonstrate which proteins of the body were being synthesized nor did they address the issue of changes in body musculature during times of bodybuilding. The results do, however, provide investigators with a potential reason to conduct such studies to determine if this effect could mean that casein is a better protein source for bodybuilders than whey. No other proteins have been similarly compared, which makes it impossible to assess the efficacy of other proteins (such as egg, soy, etc.) in comparison to whey or casein.

Wild oats (*Avena sativa*) have been marketed for their ability improve circulating testosterone concentrations due to their sterol content; however, there is no evidence to support the conversion of plant sterols to testosterone in the human body.[173] Wild oat supplementation has been used as a natural aphrodisiac and strength enhancer by men and women without any published scientific support. No adverse effects on health have been reported, but there is no solid research upon which to base a recommendation for supplementation in athletes.

Y

Yeast There are many types of yeast used in food production and available in the diet. Most individuals are familiar with baker's yeast, used as a leavening agent in baked goods. Brewer's yeast is a byproduct of the production of beer and is also available as a dietary supplement. Some producers market nutritional yeast, so called for its development as a dietary supplement. The typical yeast used to produce these varieties is *Saccharomyces cerevisiae*. As dietary supplements, yeasts are pasteurized prior to consumption. Yeasts are typically high in nutrients including proteins, vitamins, minerals, and other potentially beneficial compounds including carbohydrates, fibers, and so forth.

Yeast is often touted as an ergogenic aid due to its high content of many vital nutrients. Research to support those claims is lacking, however. Although yeasts are nutrient-dense substances, in a normally nourished athlete, the addition of yeast to the diet is unlikely to enhance performance.

Yohimbine is an extract from from the bark of *Pausinystalia yohimbe* tree. Yohimbine is considered the active ingredient of this extract. This chemical has reported functional properties as an alpha-2-antagonist. When alpha-2 receptors are blocked, lipolysis of adipose cells can be stimulated via increased action of catecholamines. Stimulation of lipolysis increases the free fatty acid concentration of the serum, which can shift fuel metabolism from carbohydrate use to fat use, thus sparing carbohydrates.[93]

While research assessing the ergogenic potential of yohimbe is lacking, yohimbine has been evaluated to some extent regarding its effect on metabolism. Stimulation of adipocyte lipolysis has been detected in cellular research.[394] Oral supplementation of yohimbine may elevate serum concentration of glycerol and free fatty acids, which also suggests that lipolysis is stimulated.[395] A dose of 0.2 mg of yohimbine per kg of body weight is considered necessary for alterations in lipolysis.

The pure form of yohimbine is currently available only through a prescription. As such it is usually prescribed by physicians to address problems related to impotence. Safety concerns stem from the fact that alpha-2-receptors are located in critical tissues including the heart and lungs; thus, alterations can potentially shift vital processes. Side effects such as panic, clumsiness, confusion, chills, nausea, and tremors have

Y–Z

been reported, but a recent review suggests that the risk of side effects are low when yohimbine is administered at common doses.[396]

Young athletes In general, the nutritional principles that can optimize performance in adults should also apply to children. However, two overriding issues should be considered with young athletes. First, since children are growing, their nutritional needs are foremost in sports dietetics. All essential nutrients must be consumed at their needed levels, but adequate energy and protein are extremely critical for normal growth. The other major consideration for children is safety. Supplements that pose even the potential for minor risk should not be recommended for young athletes. A registered dietitian should be consulted before initiating questionable dietary practices in children.

Z

Zinc is a micromineral that participates in many vital functions within the body. Dietary zinc is obtained by a variety of foods including protein rich foods such as meat, fish, poultry, and oysters, as well as whole grains and some vegetables. Some of zinc's functions include involvement with protein synthesis, energy metabolism, sexual maturation, immune function, and taste. Many of the roles of zinc are carried out through its function as a cofactor for enzymes. Zinc deficiency produces an array of problems including abnormal growth and reproduction, poor wound healing, dysgeusia (abnormal taste), decreased immune function, and various other problems.

Zinc supplements have been promoted by some for their potential to enhance muscle mass and strength. Some research has indicated that zinc supplementation improved strength in one of three isokinetic tests and also improved isometric but not isokinetic endurance.[397] The researchers suggested that zinc may have enhanced performance by improving function of the lactate dehydrogenase system. Although the data in that study were not entirely consistent, surprisingly little research has been conducted to further examine this potential role of zinc.

Zinc has also received attention due to its role in immune function. Since research suggests that athletes are more susceptible to infections, particularly during periods of overtraining, some have speculated that zinc supplementation may be beneficial. Valid research to support or reject this possibility is needed.

Y–Z

References

1. Goldberg, A. and Odessey, R., Oxidation of amino acid by diaphragms from fed and fasted rats, *Am. J. Physiol.*, 223:1384, 1972.
2. White, T.P. and Brooks, G.A., [U-14C]Glucose, -alanine, and -leucine oxidation in rats at rest and two intensities of running, *Am. J. Physiol.*, 240:E155, 1981.
3. Wolff, J. et al., Alanine decreases the protein requirements of infants with inborn errors of amino acid metabolism, *J. Neurogenet.*, 2:41–49, 1985.
4. Kelts, D. et. al., Studies on requirements for amino acids of infants with disorders of amino acid metabolism. I. Effect of alanine, *Pediatr. Res.*, 19:86, 1985.
5. Bodamer, O.A.F., Halliday, D., and Leonard, J.V., The effects of L-alanine supplementation in late-onset glycogen storage disease type II, *Neurology*, 55:710, 2000.
6. Kern, M., Klein, J., and Nyhan, W.L., unpublished data, 2004.
7. Mukamal, K. et al., Roles of drinking pattern and type of alcohol consumed in coronary heart disease in men, *N. Engl. J. Med.*, 348:109, 2003.
8. Ziegenfuss, T.N. and Kerrigan D.J., Safety and efficacy of prohormone administration in men, *J. Ex. Physiol.*, 2, abstract, 1999.
9. King, D.S. et al., Effect of oral androstenedione on serum testosterone and adaptations to resistance training in young men: a randomized controlled trial, *JAMA*, 281:2020, 1999.
10. Van Gammeren, D., Falk, D., and Antonio, J., The effects of supplementation with 19-nor-4-androstene-3,17-dione and 19-nor-4-androstene-3,17-diol on body composition and athletic performance in previously weight-trained male athletes, *Eur. J. Appl. Physiol.*, 84:426, 2001.
11. Rasmussen, B.B. et al., Androstenedione does not stimulate muscle protein anabolism in young healthy men, *J. Clin. Endocrinol. Metab.*, 85:55, 2000.
12. Wallace, M.B. et al., Effects of dehydroepiandrosterone vs. androstenedione supplementation in men, *Med. Sci. Sports Exerc.*, 31:1788, 1999.
13. Earnest, C.P. et al., *In vivo* 4-androstene-3,17-dione and 4-androstene-3 beta,17 beta-diol supplementation in young men, *Eur. J. Appl. Physiol.*, 81:229, 2000.
14. Leder, B.Z. et al., Oral androstenedione administration and serum testosterone concentrations in young men, *JAMA*, 283:779, 2000.
15. Powers, S.K., Ji, L.L., and Leeuwenburgh, C., Exercise training-induced alterations in skeletal muscle antioxidant capacity: a brief review, *Med. Sci. Sports Exerc.*, 31:987, 1999.
16. McBride, J. et al., Effect of resistance exercise on free radical production, *Med. Sci. Sports Exerc.*, 30:67, 1998.

17. Alessio, H.M., Exercise-induced oxidative stress, *Med. Sci. Sports Exerc.*, 25:218, 1993.

18. Urso, M.L. and Clarkson, P.M., Oxidative stress, exercise, and antioxidant supplementation, *Toxicol.*, 189:41, 2003.

19. Antonio, J. and Stout, J.R., *Sports Supplements*, Lippincott Williams & Wilkins: Philadelphia, 2001.

20. Tiidus, P.M., Pushkarenko, J., and Houston, M.E., Lack of antioxidant adaptation to short-term aerobic training in human muscle, *Am. J. Physiol.*, 271:R832, 1996.

21. Powers, S.K. et al., Dietary antioxidants and exercise, *J. Sports Sci.*, 22:81, 2004.

22. Gey, G.O., Cooper, K.H., and Bottenberg, R.A., Effect of ascorbic acid on endurance performance and athletic injury, *JAMA*, 211:105, 1970.

23. Howald, H., Segesser, B., and Korner, W.F., Ascorbic acid and athletic performance, *Ann. N.Y. Acad. Sci.*, 258:458, 1974.

24. Keith, R.E. and Merrill, E., The effects of vitamin C on maximum grip strength and muscular endurance, *J. Sports Med.*, 23:253, 1983.

25. Keren, G. and Epstein, Y., The effect of high dosage vitamin C intake on aerobic and anaerobic capacity, *J. Sports Med.*, 20:145, 1980.

26. Buzina, R. and Suboticanec, K., Vitamin C and physical working capacity, *Int. J. Vitam. Nutr. Res. Suppl.*, 27:157, 1985.

27. Van der Beek, E.J. et al., Controlled vitamin C restriction and physical performance in volunteers, *J. Am. Coll. Nutr.*, 9:332, 1990.

28. Kaminski, M. and Boal, R., An effect of ascorbic acid on delayed-onset muscle soreness, *Pain*, 50:317, 1992.

29. Thompson, D. et al., Muscle soreness and damage parameters after prolonged intermittent shuttle-running following acute vitamin C supplementation, *Int. J. Sports Med.*, 22:68, 2001.

30. Jakeman, P. and Maxwell, S., Effect of antioxidant vitamin supplementation on muscle function after eccentric exercise, *Eur. J. Appl. Physiol.*, 67:426, 1993.

31. Sharman, I.M., Down, M.G., and Norgan, N.G., The effects of vitamin E and training on physiological function and athletic performance in adolescent swimmers, *Br. J. Nutr.*, 26:265, 1971.

32. Lawrence, J.D. et al., The effect of alpha-tocopherol (vitamin E) and pyridoxine HCL (vitamin B_6) on the swimming endurance of trained swimmers, *J. Am. Coll. Health Assoc.*, 23:219, 1975.

33. Lawrence, J.D. et al., Effects of alpha-tocopherol acetate on the swimming endurance of trained swimmers, *Am. J. Clin. Nutr.*, 28:205, 1975.

34. Shephard, R.J. et al., Vitamin E, exercise, and the recovery from physical activity, *Eur. J. Appl. Physiol.*, 33:119, 1974.

35. Sharman, I.M., Down, M.G., and Norgan, N.G., The effects of vitamin E on physiological function and athletic performance of trained swimmers, *J. Sports Med.*, 16:215, 1976.

36. Helgheim, I. et al., The effects of vitamin E on serum enzyme levels following heavy exercise, *Eur. J. Appl. Physiol.*, 40:283, 1979.

37. Itoh, H. et al., Vitamin E supplementation attenuates leakage of enzymes following six successive days of running training, *Int. J. Sports Med.*, 21:369, 2000.
38. Kanter, M.M., Nolte, L.A., and Holloszy, J.D., Effects of an antioxidant vitamin mixture on lipid peroxidation at rest and postexercise, *J. Appl. Physiol.*, 74:965, 1993.
39. Sen, C.K. and Goldfarb, A.H., Antioxidants and physical exercise, in *Handbook of Oxidants and Antioxidants in Exercise*, Sen, C.K., Ed., Elsevier: Amsterdam, 297, 2000.
40. Tessier, F. et al., Selenium and training effects on the glutathione system and aerobic performance, *Med. Sci. Sports Exerc.*, 27:390, 1995.
41. Malm, C. et al., Supplementation with ubiquinone-10 causes cellular damage during intense exercise, *Acta Physiol. Scand.*, 157:511, 1996.
42. Laaksonen, R. et al., Ubiquinone supplementation and exercise capacity in trained young and older men, *Eur. J. Appl. Physiol.*, 72:95, 1995.
43. Chromiak, J. and Antonio, J., Use of amino acids as growth-hormone releasing agents by athletes, *Nutrition*, 18:657, 2002.
44. Ahlborg, B., Effect of potassium-magnesium-aspartate on the capacity for prolonged exercise in man, *Acta Phyiol. Scand.*, 74:238, 1968.
45. Kendrick, Z.V. et al., Potassium aspartate treatment: effects on blood ammonia, urea and exercise to exhaustion, *Med. Sci. Sports Exerc.*, 8:70, 1976.
46. Wesson, M.L. et al., Effects of oral administration of aspartic acid salts on endurance capacity of trained athletes, *Res. Q. Exerc. Sport*, 59:234, 1988.
47. Consolazio, C.F. et al., Effects of aspartic acid salts (Mg and K) on physical performance of men, *J. Appl. Physiol.*, 19:257, 1964.
48. Maughan, R.L. and Sadler, D.J.M., The effects of oral administration of salts of aspartic acid on the metabolic response to prolonged exhausting exercise in man, *Int. J. Sports Med.*, 4:119, 1983.
49. DeHann, A., Van Doorn, J.E., and Westra, H.G., Effects of potassium + magnesium aspartate on muscle metabolism and force development during short intensive static exercise, *Int. J. Sports Med.*, 6:44, 1985.
50. Tuttle, J.L. et al., Effect of acute potassium-magnesium aspartate supplementation on ammonia concentrations during and after resistance training, *Int. J. Sport Nutr.*, 5:102, 1995.
51. Tripplett, N.T. et al., Effects of aspartic acid salts on fatigue parameters during weight training exercise and recovery, *J. Appl. Sport Sci. Res.*, 4:141, 1990.
52. Frankenfield, D.C., Muth, E.R., and Rowe, W.A., The Harris-Benedict studies of human basal metabolism: history and limitations, *J. Am. Diet. Assoc.*, 98:439, 1998.
53. Speakman, J.R. and Selman, C., Physical activity and resting metabolic rate, *Proc. Nutr. Soc.*, 62:621, 2003.
54. Williams, M.H., *Nutrition for Health, Fitness & Sport*, 7th ed., McGraw-Hill: New York, 273, 2004.
55. Bendich, A., From 1989 to 2001: what have we learned about the "biological actions of beta-carotene"? *J. Nutr.*, 134:225S, 2004.

56. Robert, J. and Burri, B., Oxidative damage and defense, *Am. J. Clin. Nutr.*, 63:985S, 1996.

57. Marchioli, R. et al., Antioxidant vitamins and prevention of cardiovascular disease: epidemiological and clinical trial data, *Lipids*, 36:S53, 2001.

58. Hasnain, B.I. and Mooradian, A.D., Recent trials of antioxidant therapy: what should we be telling our patients? *Cleve. Clin. J. Med.*, 71:327, 2004.

59. Johnson, L.J., Meacham, S.L., and Kruskall, L.J., The antioxidants-vitamin C, vitamin E, selenium, and carotenoids, *J. Agromed.*, 9:65, 2003.

60. Tran, T.L., Antioxidant supplements to prevent heart disease, *Postgrad. Med.*, 109:109, 2001.

61. Powers, S.K. and Hamilton, K., Antioxidants and exercise, *Clin. Sports Med.*, 18:525, 1999.

62. Nissen, S. et al., Effect of leucine metabolite beta-hydroxy-beta-methylbutryate on muscle metabolism during resistance-exercise training, *J. Appl. Physiol.*, 81:2095, 1996.

63. McArdle, W., Katch, F., and Katch, V., *Sports and Exercise Nutrition*, Lippincott Williams and Wilkins: Philadelphia, chap. 12, 1999.

64. Nieman, D., *Fitness and Sports Medicine*, Bull Publishing: Palo Alto, CA, 1990.

65. Williams, C. and Bale, P., Bias and limits of agreement between hydrodensitometry, bioelectrical impedance and skinfold calipers measures of percentage body fat, *Eur. J. Appl. Physiol.*, 77:271, 1998.

66. Segal, K., Use of bioelectrical impedance analysis measurements as an evaluation for participating in sports, *Am. J. Clin. Nutr.*, 64:469S, 1996.

67. Singh, A., Moses, F.M., and Deuster, P.A., Chronic multivitamin-mineral supplementation does not enhance physical performance, *Med. Sci. Sports Exerc.*, 24;726, 1992.

68. Telford, R.D. et al., The effect of 7 to 8 months of vitamin/mineral supplementation on athletic performance, *Int. J. Sport Nutr.*, 2:135, 1992.

69. Brooks, G. et al., *Exercise Physiology: Human Bioenergetics and its Applications*, 3rd ed., McGraw-Hill: New York, 2000.

70. McArdle, W., Katch, F., and Katch, V., *Sports and Exercise Nutrition*, Lippincott Williams & Wilkins: Philadelphia, chap. 5, 1999.

71. Teegarden, D. et al., Peak spine and femoral neck bone mass in young women, *J. Bone Min. Res.*, 10:711, 1995.

72. Lin, Y.C. et al., Peak spine and femoral neck bone mass in young women, *Bone*, 32:546, 2003.

73. McArdle, W., Katch, F., and Katch, V., *Sports and Exercise Nutrition*, Lippincott Williams & Wilkins: Philadelphia, chap. 2, 1999.

74. Cromer, B. and Harel, Z., Adolescents: at increased risk for osteoporosis? *Clin. Ped.*, 39:565, 2000.

75. Sheth, P., Osteoporosis and exercise, *Mount Sinai J. Med.*, 66:197, 1999.

76. Keen, A.D. and Drinkwater, B.L., Irreversible bone loss in former amenorrheic athletes, *Osteoporosis Int.*, 7:311, 1997.

77. Nattiv, A. and Lynch, L., The female athlete triad: managing an acute risk to long-term health, *Phys. Sportsmed.*, 22:60, 1994.

78. Nielsen, F.H., The justification for providing dietary guidance for the nutritional intake of boron, *Biol. Trace Elem. Res.*, 66:319, 1998.

79. Farrando, A. and Green, N., The effect of boron supplementation on lean body mass, plasma testosterone levels, and strength in male bodybuilders, *Int. J. Sport Nutr.*, 3:140, 1993.

80. Davis, J.M., Alderson, N.L., and Welsh, R.S., Serotonin and central nervous system fatigue: nutritional considerations, *Am. J. Clin. Nutr.*, 72:573S, 2000.

81. Madsen, K. et al., Effects of glucose, glucose plus branched-chain amino acids, or placebo on bike performance over 100 km, *J. Appl. Physiol.*, 81:2644, 1996.

82. Mittleman, K.D., Ricci, M.R., and Bailey, S.P., Branched-chain amino acids prolong exercise during heat stress in men and women, *Med. Sci. Sports Exerc.*, 30:83, 1998.

83. Blomstrand, E. et al., Administration of branched-chain amino acids during sustained exercise—effects on performance and on plasma concentration of some amino acids, *Eur. J. Appl. Physiol.*, 63:83, 1991.

84. Blomstrand, E., Ekblom, S., and Newsholme, E.A., Influence of ingesting a solution of branched-chain amino acids on plasma and muscle concentrations of amino acids during prolonged submaximal exercise, *Nutrition*, 12:485, 1996.

85. Blomstrand, E. et al., Effect of branched-chain amino acid and carbohydrate supplementation on the exercise-induced change in plasma and muscle concentration of amino acids in human subjects, *Acta Physiol. Scand.*, 153:87, 1995.

86. Van Hall, G., Raaymakers, J.S., Saris, W.H., and Wagenmakers, A.J., Ingestion of branched-chain amino acids and tryptophan during sustained exercise in man: failure to affect performance, *J. Physiol.*, 486:789, 1995.

87. Armstrong, L., Caffeine, body fluid-electrolyte balance and exercise performance, *Int. J. Sport Nutr. Exerc. Metab.*, 21:189, 2002.

88. McArdle, W., Katch, F., and Katch, V., *Sports and Exercise Nutrition*, Lippincott Williams & Wilkins: Philadelphia, chap. 10, 1999.

89. Maughan, R., King, D., and Lea, T., Dietary supplements, *J. Sports Sci.*, 22:95, 2004.

90. Costill, D.L., Dalsky, G.P., and Fink, W.J., Effects of caffeine ingestion on metabolism and exercise performance, *Med. Sci. Sports*, 10:155, 1978.

91. Ivy, J.L. et al., Influence of caffeine and carbohydrate feedings on endurance performance, *Med. Sci. Sports*, 11:6, 1979.

92. Graham, T. and Spriet, T., Performance and metabolic responses to a high caffeine dose during prolonged exercise, *J. Appl. Physiol.*, 85:883, 1991.

93. Hargreaves, M., Kiens, B., and Richter, E.A., Effect of increased plasma free fatty acid concentrations on muscle metabolism in exercising men, *J. Appl. Physiol.*, 70:194, 1991.

94. Pasman, W.J. et al., The effect of different dosages of caffeine on endurance performance time, *Int. J. Sports Med.*, 16:225, 1995.

95. MacIntosh, B.R. and Wright, B.M., Caffeine ingestion and performance of a 1,500-meter swim, *Can. J. Appl. Physiol.*, 20:168, 1995.

96. Williams, M.H., *Nutrition for Health, Fitness & Sport*, 7th ed., McGraw-Hill: New York, chap. 4, 2002.
97. Jacobs, K.A. and Sherman, W.M., The efficacy of carbohydrate supplementation and chronic high carbohydrate diets for improving endurance performance, *Int. J. Sport Nutr.*, 9:92–115, 1999.
98. Sherman, W.M. et al., Effects of 4 h pre-exercise carbohydrate feedings on cycling performance, *Med. Sci. Sports Exerc.*, 21:598, 1989.
99. Sherman, W.M., Peden, M.C., and Wright, D.A., Carbohydrate feedings 1 hour before exercise improves cycling performance, *Am. J. Clin. Nutr.*, 54:866, 1991.
100. Below, P.R. et al., Fluid and carbohydrate ingestion independently improve performance during 1 hour of intense exercise, *Med. Sci. Sports Exerc.*, 27:200, 1995.
101. Coyle, E.F. et al., Carbohydrate feeding during prolonged strenuous exercise can delay fatigue, *J. Appl. Physiol.*, 55:230, 1983.
102. Wright, D.A., Sherman, W.M., and Dernbach, A.R., Carbohydrate feedings before, during, or in combination improves cycling endurance performance, *J. Appl. Physiol.*, 71:1082, 1991.
103. Ivy, J.L. et al., Effect of a carbohydrate–protein supplement on endurance performance during exercise of varying intensity, *Int. J. Sport Nutr. Exerc. Metab.*, 13:382, 2003.
104. Sherman, W.M. et al., Dietary carbohydrate, muscle glycogen, and exercise performance during 7 d of training, *Am. J. Clin. Nutr.*, 57:27, 1993.
105. Lambert, E.V. et al., Enhanced endurance in trained cyclists during moderate intensity exercise following 2 weeks adaptation to a high fat diet, *Eur. J. Appl. Physiol.*, 69:287, 1994.
106. Ivy, J.L. et al., Muscle glycogen synthesis after exercise: effect of time of carbohydrate ingestion, *J. Appl. Physiol.*, 6:1490, 1988.
107. Van Hall, G., Shirreffs, S., and Calbet, J., Muscle glycogen resynthesis during recovery from cycle exercise: no effect of additional protein ingestion, *J. Appl. Physiol.*, 88:1631, 2000.
108. Van Loon, L. et al., Maximizing postexercise muscle glycogen synthesis: carbohydrate supplementation and the application of amino acid or protein hydrolysate mixtures, *Am. J. Clin. Nutr.*, 72:106, 2000.
109. Rasmussen, B.B. et al., An oral essential amino acid-carbohydrate supplement enhances muscle protein anabolism after resistance exercise, *J. Appl. Physiol.*, 88:386, 2000.
110. DeMarco, H.M. et al., Pre-exercise carbohydrate meals: application of glycemic index, *Med. Sci. Sports Exerc.*, 31:164, 1999.
111. Kirwan, J.P., O'Gorman, D., and Evans, W.J., A moderate glycemic meal before endurance exercise can enhance performance, *J. Appl. Physiol.*, 84:53, 1998.
112. Tarnopolsky, M.A. et al., Carbohydrate loading and metabolism during exercise in men and women, *J. Appl. Physiol.*, 78:1360, 1995.
113. Pizza, F.X. et al., A carbohydrate loading regimen improves high intensity, short duration exercise performance, *Int. J. Sports Med.*, 5:110, 1995.

114. Kanter, M.M. and Williams, M.H., Antioxidants, carnitine, and choline as putative ergogenic aids, *Int. J. Sport Nutr.*, 5:S120, 1995.

115. Lombard, K.A. et al., Carnitine status of lactoovovegetarians and strict vegetarian adults and children, *Am. J. Clin. Nutr.*, 50:301, 1989.

116. Rebouche, C.J. and Seim, H., Carnitine metabolism and its regulation in microorganisms and mammals, *Annu. Rev. Nutr.*, 18:39, 1998.

117. Arenas, J. et al., Carnitine in muscle, serum, and urine of nonprofessional athletes; effects of physical exercise, training, and L-carnitine administration, *Muscle Nerve*, 14:598, 1991.

118. Daily, J.W. and Sachan, D.S., Choline supplementation alters carnitine homeostasis in humans and guinea pigs, *J. Nutr.*, 125:1938, 1995.

119. Barnett, C. et al., Effect of L-carnitine supplementation on muscle and blood carnitine content and lactate accumulation during high-intensity spring cycling, *Int. J. Sport Nutr.*, 4:280, 1994.

120. Soop, M. et al., Influence of supplementation on muscle substrate and carnitine metabolism during exercise, *J. Appl. Physiol.*, 64(6):2394, 1988.

121. Vukovich, M., Costill, D., and Fink, W., L-carnitine supplementation: Effect on muscle carnitine content and glycogen utilization during exercise, *Med. Sci. Sports Exerc.*, 26:1122, 1994.

122. Gorostiagam E.M., Maurer, C.A., and Eclache, J.P., Decrease in respiratory quotient during exercise following L-carnitine supplementation, *Int. J. Sports Med.*, 10:169, 1989.

123. Kasper, C.M. et al., L-carnitine supplementation and running performance, *Med. Sci. Sports Exerc.*, 26:S39, 1994.

124. Decombaz, J. et al., Effect of L-carnitine on submaximal exercise metabolism after depletion of muscle glycogen, *Med. Sci. Sports Exerc.*, 25(6):733, 1993.

125. Colombani, P. et al., Effects of L-carnitine supplementation on physical performance and energy metabolism of endurance-trained athletes: A double blind cross-over field study, *Eur. J. Appl. Phys.*, 73:434, 1996.

126. Greig, C. et al., The effect of oral supplementation with L-carnitine on maximum and submaximum exercise capacity, *Eur. J. Appl. Physiol.*, 56:457, 1985.

127. Oyono-Enguelle, S. et al., Prolonged submaximal exercise and L-carnitine in humans, *Eur. J. Appl. Physiol.*, 58:53, 1988.

128. Trappe, S.W. et al., The effects of L-carnitine supplementation on performance during interval swimming, *Int. J. Sports Med.*, 15(4):181, 1994.

129. Wachter, S. et al., Long-term administration of L-carnitine to humans: effect on skeletal muscle carnitine content and physical performance, *Clin. Chim. Acta*, 318:51, 2002.

130. Wyss, V., Ganzit, G.P., and Rienzi, A., Effects of L-carnitine administration on VO_{2max} and the aerobic-anaerobic threshold in normoxia and acute hypoxia, *Eur. J. Appl. Physiol.*, 60:1, 1990.

131. Marconi, C. et al., Effects of L-carnitine loading on the aerobic and anaerobic performance of endurance athletes, *Eur. J. Appl. Physiol.*, 54:131, 1985.

132. Cha, Y.S. et al., Effects of carnitine coingested caffeine on carnitine metabolism and endurance capacity in athletes, *J. Nutr. Sci. Vitaminol.*, 47:378, 2001.

133. Durstine, J.L. and Haskell, W.L., Effects of exercise training on plasma lipids and lipoproteins, *Exerc. Sports Sci. Rev.*, 22:477, 1994.

134. Paffenbarger, R.S. et al., The association of changes in physical activity level and other lifestyle characteristics with mortality among men, *New Eng. J. Med.*, 328:538, 1993.

135. Brown, R.C. and Cox, C.M., Effects of high fat versus high carbohydrate diets on plasma lipids and lipoproteins in endurance athletes, *Med. Sci. Sports Exerc.*, 30:1677, 1998.

136. Leddy, J. et al., Effect of a high or a low fat diet on cardiovascular risk factors in male and female runners, *Med. Sci. Sports Exerc.*, 29:17, 1997.

137. Evans, G.W., The effect of chromium picolinate on insulin controlled parameters in humans, *Int. J. Biosoc. Med. Res.*, 11:163, 1989.

138. Hasten, D.L. et al., Effects of chromium picolinate on beginning weight training students, *Int. J. Sport Nutr.*, 2:343, 1992.

139. Trent, L.K. and Thieding-Cancel, D., Effects of chromium picolinate on body composition, *J. Sports Med. Phys. Fitness*, 35:273, 1995.

140. Lukaski, H.C. et al., Chromium supplementation and resistance training: effects on body composition, strength, and trace element status of men, *Am. J. Clin. Nutr.*, 63:954, 1996.

141. Walker, L.S. et al., Chromium picolinate effects on body composition and muscular performance in wrestlers, *Med. Sci. Sports Exerc.*, 30:1730, 1998.

142. Lefavi, R.G. et. al., Efficacy of chromium supplementation in athletes: emphasis on anabolism, *Int. J. Sport Nutr.*, 2:111, 1992.

143. Hallmark, M.A. et al., Effects of chromium and resistance training on muscle strength and body composition, *Med. Sci. Sports Exerc.*, 28:139, 1996.

144. Campbell, W.W. et al., Effects of resistance training and chromium picolinate on body composition and skeletal muscle in older men, *J. Appl. Physiol.*, 86:29, 1999.

145. Clancy, S.P. et al., Effects of chromium picolinate supplementation on body composition, strength, and urinary chromium loss in football players, *Int. J. Sport Nutr.*, 4:142, 1994.

146. Grant, K.E. et al., Chromium and exercise training: effect on obese women, *Med. Sci. Sports Exerc.*, 29:992, 1994.

147. Cheuvront, S.N. et al., Effect of ENDUROX (on metabolic responses to submaximal exercise, *Int. J. Sport Nutr.*, 9:434, 1999.

148. Plowman, S. et al., The effects of ENDUROX (on the physiological responses to stair-stepping exercise, *Res. Q. Exerc. Sport*, 70:385, 1999.

149. Greenberg, S. and Fishman, W.H., Coenzyme Q_{10}: a new drug for cardiovascular disease, *J. Clin. Pharmacol.*, 30:596, 1990.

150. Watson, P.S. et al., Lack of effect of coenzyme Q on left ventricular function in patients with congestive heart failure, *J. Am. Coll. Cardiol.*, 33:1549, 1999.

151. Morisco, C., Trimarco, B., and Condorelli, M., Effect of coenzyme Q_{10} therapy in patients with congestive heart failure: A long-term, multicenter, randomized study, *Clin. Invest.*, 71:S134, 1993.
152. Kaikkonen, J. et al., Coenzyme Q_{10}: absorption, antioxidative properties, determinants, and plasma levels, *Free Radic. Res.*, 36:389, 2002.
153. Nielsen, A.N. et al., No effect of antioxidant supplementation in triathletes on maximal oxygen uptake, 31P-NMRS detected muscle energy metabolism and muscle fatigue, *Int. J. Sports Med.*, 20:154, 1999.
154. Weston, S.B. et al., Does exogenous coenzyme Q_{10} affect aerobic capacity in endurance athletes? *Int. J. Sport Nutr.*, 7:197, 1997.
155. Bonetti, A. et al., Effect of ubidecarenone oral treatment on aerobic power in middle-aged trained subjects, *J. Sports Med. Phys. Fitness*, 40:51, 2000.
156. Braun, B. et al., Effects of coenzyme Q_{10} supplementation on exercise performance, VO_{2max}, and lipid peroxidation in trained cyclists, *Int. J. Sport Nutr.*, 1:353, 1991.
157. Malm, C. et al., Effects of ubiquinone-10 supplementation and high intensity training on physical performance in humans, *Acta Physiol. Scand.*, 161:379, 1997.
158. Ylikoski, T. et al., The effect of coenzyme Q_{10} on the exercise performance of cross-country skiers, *Mol. Aspects Med.*, 18:S283, 1997.
159. Coombes, J.S. et al., Dose effects of oral bovine colostrum on physical work capacity in cyclists, *Med. Sci. Sport Exerc.*, 34:1184, 2002.
160. Hofman, Z. et al., The effect of bovine colostrum supplementation on exercise performance in elite field hockey players, *Int. J. Sport Nutr. Exerc. Metab.*, 12:461, 2002.
161. Antonio, J., Sanders, M.S., and Van Gammeren, D., The effects of bovine colostrum supplementation on body composition and exercise performance in active men and women, *Nutrition*, 17:243, 2001.
162. Buckley, J.D. et al., Bovine colostrum supplementation during endurance running training improves recovery, but not performance, *J. Sci. Med. Sport*, 5:65, 2002.
163. Brinkworth, G.D. et al., Oral bovine colostrum supplementation enhances buffer capacity but not rowing performance in elite female rowers, *Int. J. Sport Nutr. Exerc. Metab.*, 12:349, 2002.
164. Pariza, M.W. et al., Formation and action of anticarcinogenic fatty acids, *Adv. Exp. Med. Biol.*, 289:269, 1991.
165. Ritzenthaler, K.L. et al., Estimation of conjugated linoleic acid intake by written dietary assessment methodologies underestimates actual intake evaluated by food duplicate methodology, *J. Nutr.*, 131:1548, 2001.
166. Lowery, L.M. et al., *Med. Sci. Sports Exerc.*, 30:S182, 1998.
167. Park, Y. et al., Effect of conjugated linoleic acid on body composition in mice, *Lipids*, 32:853, 1997.
168. Kreider, R.B. et al., Effects of conjugated linoleic acid supplementation during resistance training on body composition, bone density, strength, and selected hematological markers, *J. Strength Cond. Res.*, 16:325, 2002.

169. Zambell, K.L. et al., Conjugated linoleic acid supplementation in humans: effects on body composition and energy expenditure, *Lipids*, 35:777, 2000.

170. Zambell, K.L., Horn, W.F., and Keim, N.L., Conjugated linoleic acid supplementation in humans: effects on fatty acid and glycerol kinetics, *Lipids*, 36:767, 2001.

171. Houseknecht, K.L. et al., Dietary conjugated linoleic acid normalizes impaired glucose tolerance in the Zucker diabetic fatty fa/fa rat, *Biochem. Biophys. Res. Comm.*, 244:678, 1998.

172. Lukaski, H., Micronutrients (magnesium, zinc, and copper): Are mineral supplements needed for athletes? *Int. J. Sport Nutr.*, 5:S74, 1995.

173. Bucci, L., Selected herbals and human exercise performance, *Am. J. Clin. Nutr.*, 72:624s, 2000.

174. Parcell, A.C. et al., Cordyceps Sinensis (CordyMax Cs-4) supplementation does not improve endurance exercise performance, *Int. J. Sport Nutr. Exerc. Metab.*, 14:236, 2004.

175. Antonio, J. and Stout, J.R., *Sports Supplements*, Lippincott Williams & Wilkins: Philadelphia, chap. 3, 2001.

176. Burke, D.G. et al., Effect of creatine and weight training on muscle creatine and performance in vegetarians, *Med. Sci. Sports Exerc.*, 35:1946, 2003.

177. Lukaszuk, J.M. et al., Effect of creatine supplementation and a lacto-ovo-vegetarian diet on muscle creatine concentration, *Int. J. Sport Nutr. Exerc. Metab.*, 12:336, 2002.

178. Balsom, P., Soderland, K., and Ekblom, B., Creatine in humans with special reference to creatine supplementation, *Sports Med.*, 18:268, 1994.

179. Lawrence, M. and Kirby, D., Nutrition and sports supplements: fact or fiction? *J. Clin. Gastroenter.*, 35:299, 2002.

180. Mujika, I. et al., Creatine supplementation does not improve sprint performance in competitive swimmers, *Med. Sci. Sports Exerc.*, 28:1435, 1996.

181. Rockwell, J.A., Rankin, J.W., and Toderico, B., Creatine supplementation affects muscle creatine during energy restriction, *Med. Sci. Sports Exerc.*, 33:61, 2001.

182. Volek, J.S. et al., Performance and muscle fiber adaptations to creatine supplementation and heavy resistance training, *Med. Sci. Sports Exerc.*, 31:1147, 1999.

183. Willoughby, D.S. and Rosene, J., Effects of oral creatine and resistance training on myosin heavy chain expression, *Med. Sci. Sports Exerc.*, 33:1674, 2001.

184. Williams, M.H. and Branch, J.D., Creatine supplementation and exercise performance: an update, *J. Am. Coll. Nutr.*, 17:216, 1998.

185. Kreider, E.B., Creatine supplementation in exercise and sport. In: Driskell, J. and Wolinsky, I. (Eds.), *Energy-Yielding Macronutrients and Energy Metabolism in Sports Nutrition*, CRC Press: Boca Raton, FL, 1999, 213.

186. Williams, M.H., Kreider, R., and Branch, J.D., *Creatine: The Power Supplement*, Human Kinetics Publishers: Champaign, IL, 1999.

187. Kreider, R.B., Effects of creatine supplementation on performance and training adaptations, *Mol. Cell Biochem.*, 244:89, 2003.

188. Gill, N.D., Hall, R.D., and Blazevich, A.J., Creatine serum is not as effective as creatine powder for improving cycle sprint performance in competitive male team-sport athletes, *J. Strength Cond. Res.*, 18:272, 2004.

189. Balsom, P. et al, Creatine supplementation per se does not enhance endurance exercise performance, *Acta Physiol. Scand.*, 149:521, 1993.

190. Rawson, E.S. and Volek, J.S., Effects of creatine supplementation and resistance training on muscle strength and weightlifting performance, *J. Strength Cond. Res.*, 17:822, 2003.

191. Kern, M. et al., Physiological response to exercise in the heat following creatine supplementation, *J. Exerc. Physiol.*, 4:18, 2001.

192. Volek, J.S. et al., Physiological responses to short-term exercise in the heat after creatine loading, *Med. Sci. Sports Exerc.*, 33:1101, 2001.

193. Vanderberie, F.B., Vandeneynde, B.M., Vandenberghe, K., et al., Effect of creatine on endurance capacity and sprint power in cyclists, *Int. J. Sports Med.*, 8:2055, 1998.

194. Kreider, R.B., Ferreira, M., and Wilson, M., Effects of creatine supplementation on body composition, strength, and sprint performance, *Med. Sci. Sports Exerc.*, 30:73, 1998.

195. Morales, A.J. et al., The effects of six months' treatment with 100 mg daily dose of dehydroepiandrosterone (DHEA) on circulating sex steroids, body composition and muscle strength in age-advanced men and women, *Clin. Endocrinol.*, 49:421, 1998.

196. Morales, A.J. et al., Effects of replacement doses of dehydroepiandrosterone in men and women of advancing age, *J. Clin. Endocrinol. Metab.*, 78:1360, 1994.

197. Brown, G.A. et al., Effect of oral DHEA on serum testosterone and adaptations to resistance training in young men, *J. Appl. Physiol.*, 87:2274, 1999.

198. Wallace, M.B. et al., Effects of dehydroepiandrosterone vs. androstenedione supplementation in men, *Med. Sci. Sports Exerc.*, 31:1788, 1999.

199. Butterfield, G., Ergogenic aids: evaluating sport nutrition products, *Int. J. Sport Nutr.*, 6:191, 1996.

200. Fairburn, C.G., Atypical eating disorders. In *Eating Disorders and Obesity: A Comprehensive Textbook*, Fairburn, C. and Brownell, K.D., Eds., 2nd ed., Guilford Press: New York, 2001.

201. Schwartz, D., Thompson, M., and Johnson, C., Anorexia nervosa and bulimia: the socio-cultural context, *Int. J. Eating Dis.*, 1:20, 1982.

202. *American Psychiatric Association, Diagnostic and Statistical Manual of Mental Disorders (DSM-IV)*, 4th ed., Washington, D.C., 1994.

203. Otis, C.L. et al., American College of Sports Medicine position stand: the female athlete triad, *Med. Sci. Sports Exerc.*, 29:i, 1997.

204. Burckes-Miller, M. and Black, D., Male and female college athletes: prevalence of anorexia nervosa and bulimia nervosa, *Ath. Train.*, 23:137, 1988.

205. Petrie, T.A., Disordered eating in female collegiate gymnasts: prevalence and personality/attitudinal correlates, *J. Sport Exerc. Psychol.*, 15:424, 1993.

206. Johnson, C., Powers, P.S., and Dick, R., Athletes and eating disorders: The National Collegiate Athletic Association study, *Int. J. Eating Dis.*, 26:179, 1999.

207. Sundgot-Borgen, J., Prevalence of eating disorders in elite female athletes, *Int. J. Sport Nutr.*, 3:29, 1993.

208. Pernick, Y. et al., unpublished data, 2004.

209. Williams, M.H., *Nutrition for Health, Fitness & Sport,* 7th ed., McGraw-Hill: New York, 179, 2004.

210. McArdle, W., Katch, F., and Katch, V., *Sports and Exercise Nutrition*, Lippincott Williams & Wilkins: Philadelphia, chap. 9, 1999.

211. Sawka, M. and Montain, S., Fluid and electrolyte supplementation for exercise heat stress, *Am. J. Clin. Nutr.*, 72:564s, 2000.

212. Maughan, R., Leiper, J., and Shirreffs, S., Rehydration and recovery after exercise, *Sports Sci. Exch.*, 9:3, 1996.

213. American College of Sports Medicine, American Dietetic Association, and Dietitians of Canada, Position statement: nutrition and athletic performance, *Med. Sci. Sports Exerc.*, 32:2130, 2000.

214. Williams, M.H., *Nutrition for Health, Fitness & Sport*, 7th ed., McGraw-Hill: New York, 184, 2004.

215. Kern, M., Ergogenic aids: prospecting for new terminology, *Int. J. Sport Nutr.*, 10:1, 2000.

216. Helge J.W., Wulff, B., and Kiens, B., Impact of a fat-rich diet on endurance in man: role of the dietary period, *Med. Sci. Sports Exerc.*, 30:456, 1998.

217. Lambert, E.V. et al., Enhanced endurance in trained cyclists during moderate intensity exercise following 2 weeks adaptation to a high fat diet, *Eur. J. Appl. Physiol.*, 69:287, 1994.

218. Muoio, D.M. et al., Effects of dietary fat on metabolic adjustments to maximal VO_2 and endurance in runners, *Med. Sci. Sports Exerc.*, 26:81, 1994.

219. Horvath, P.J. et al., The effects of varying dietary fat on performance and metabolism in trained male and female runners, *J. Am. Coll. Nutr.*, 19:52, 2000.

220. Helge, J.W., Richter, E.A., and Kiens, B., Interaction of training and diet on metabolism and endurance during exercise in man, *J. Physiol.*, 492:293, 1996.

221. Lambert, E.V. et al., High-fat diet versus habitual diet prior to carbohydrate loading: Effects of exercise metabolism and cycling performance, *Int. J. Sport Nutr. Exerc. Metab.*, 11:209, 2001.

222. Brown, R.C. and Cox, C.M., Effects of high fat versus high carbohydrate diets on plasma lipids and lipoproteins in endurance athletes, *Med. Sci. Sports Exerc.*, 30:1677, 1998.

223. Leddy, J. et al., Effect of a high or a low fat diet on cardiovascular risk factors in male and female runners, *Med. Sci. Sports Exerc.*, 29:17, 1997.

224. Vergauwen, L., Brouns, F., and Hespel, P., Carbohydrate supplementation improves stroke performance in tennis, *Med. Sci. Sports Exerc.*, 30:1289, 1998.

225. Beals, K.A., Brey, R.A., and Gonyou, J.B., Understanding the female athlete triad: eating disorders, amenorrhea, and osteoporosis, *J. School Health*, 69:337, 1999.

226. Donaldson, M.L., The female athlete triad, *Orthopaedic Nursing*, 22:322, 2003.

227. West, R.V., The female athlete: the triad of disordered eating, amenorrhoea and osteoporosis, *Sports Med.*, 26:63, 1998.

228. Mansfield, M.J. and Emans, S.J., Anorexia nervosa, athletics, and amenorrhea, *Ped. Clin. North Am.*, 36:533, 1989.

229. Nattiv, A. and Lynch, L., The female athlete triad: managing an acute risk to long-term health, *Phys. Sportsmed.*, 22:60, 1994.

230. Teegarden, D. et al., Peak spine and femoral neck bone mass in young women, *J. Bone Min. Res.*, 10:711, 1995.

231. Lin, Y.C. et al., Peak spine and femoral neck bone mass in young women, *Bone*, 32:546, 2003.

232. Seshadri, S. and Malhotra, S., The effect of hematinics on the physical work capacity in anemics, *Indian Ped.*, 21:529, 1984.

233. Singh, A., Moses, F.M., and Deuster, P.A., Chronic multivitamin–mineral supplementation does not enhance physical performance, *Med. Sci. Sports Exerc.*, 24:726, 1992.

234. Telford, R.D. et al., The effect of 7 to 8 months of vitamin/mineral supplementation on athletic performance, *Int. J. Sport Nutr.*, 2:135, 1992.

235. Jentjens, R.L. and Jeukendrup, A.E., Effects of pre-exercise ingestion of trehalose, galactose and glucose on subsequent metabolism and cycling performance, *Eur. J. Appl. Physiol.*, 88(4–5):459–465, 2003.

236. Leijssen, D.P. et al., Oxidation of exogenous [13C]galactose and [13C]glucose during exercise, *J. Appl. Physiol.*, 79(3):720–725, 1995.

237. Asha, S. and Vijayalakshmi, N.R., Impact of certain flavanoids on lipid profiles – potential action of garcinia cambogia flavanoids, *Phytother. Res.*, 15:395, 2001.

238. Hayamizu, K. et al., Effect of Garcinia cambogia extract on serum lepitin and insulin in mice, *Fitoterapia*, 74:267, 2003.

239. Yan, L.J., Droy-Lefaix, M.T., and Packer, L., Ginkgo biloba extract (EGb 761) protects human low density lipoproteins against oxidative modification mediated by copper, *Biochem. Biophys. Res. Comm.*, 212:360, 1995.

240. Bahrke, M.S. and Morgan, W.P., Evaluation of the ergogenic properties of ginseng, *Sports Med.*, 29(2):113–133, 2000.

241. Bucci, L.R., Dietary supplements as ergogenic aids. In *Nutrition in Exercise and Sport*, 3rd ed., Wolinsky, I., Ed., CRC Press: Boca Raton, FL, 315, 1998.

242. Engels, H.J., Fahlman, M.M., and Wirth, J.C., Effects of ginseng on secretory IgA, performance, and recovery from interval exercise, *Med. Sci. Sports Exerc.*, 35:690, 2003.

243. Engels, H.J. et al., Effects of ginseng supplementation on supramaximal exercise performance and short-term recovery, *J. Strength Cond. Res.*, 15:290, 2001.

244. Blumenthal, M., *The ABC Clinical Guide to Herbs*, American Botanical Council: Austin, TX, 217, 2003.
245. Walsh, D.E., Yaghoubian, V., and Behforooz, A., Effect of glucomannan on obese patients: a clinical study, *Int. J. Obes.*, 8:289, 1983.
246. Antonio, J. et al., The effects of high-dose glutamine ingestion on weight-lifting performance, *J. Strength Cond. Res.*, 16:157, 2002.
247. Bowtell, J.L. et al., Effect of oral glutamine on whole body carbohydrate storage during recovery from exhaustive exercise, *J. Appl. Physiol.*, 86:1770, 1999.
248. Haub, M.D. et al., Acute L-glutamine ingestion does not improve maximal effort exercise, *J. Sports Med. Phys. Fitness*, 38:240, 1998.
249. Castell, L., Glutamine supplementation *in vitro* and *in vivo*, in exercise and in immunodepression, *Sports Med.*, 33:323, 2003.
250. Burke, L.M., Collier, G.R., and Hargreaves, M., Glycemic index—-a new tool in sport nutrition? *Int. J. Sport Nutr.*, 8:401, 1998.
251. Coggan, A.R. and Coyle E.F., Carbohydrate ingestion during prolonged exercise: effects on metabolism and performance. In *Exercise and Sports Science Reviews*, Vol. 19, Holloszy, J., Ed., Williams & Wilkins: Baltimore, 1, 1991.
252. Robergs, R.A. et al., Blood glucose and glucoregulatory hormone response to solid and liquid carbohydrate ingestion during exercise, *Int. J. Sport Nutr.*, 8:70, 1998.
253. Guezennec, C.Y., Oxidation rates, complex carbohydrates and exercise, *Sports Med.*, 19:365, 1995.
254. Kern, M., Heslin, C.J., and Rezende, R.S., Metabolic and performance effects of raisins versus sports gel as preexercise feedings in cyclists, *Med. Sci. Sports Exerc.*, 36:S174, 2004.
255. DeMarco, H.M. et al., Pre-exercise carbohydrate meals: application of glycemic index, *Med. Sci. Sports Exerc.*, 31:164, 1999.
256. Thomas, D.E. et al., Plasma glucose levels after prolonged strenuous exercise correlates inversely with glycemic response to food consumed before exercise, *Int. J. Sport Nutr.*, 4:361, 1994.
257. Kirwan, J.P., O'Gorman, D., and Evans, W.J., A moderate glycemic meal before endurance exercise can enhance performance, *J. Appl. Physiol.*, 84:53, 1998.
258. Thomas, D.E., Brotherhood, J.R., and Brand, J.C., Carbohydrate feeding before exercise: effect of glycemic index, *Int. J. Sports Med.*, 12:180, 1991.
259. Febbraio, M.A. et al., Pre-exercise carbohydrate ingestion, glucose kinetics, and muscle glycogen use: effect of the glycemic index, *J. Appl. Physiol.*, 89:1845, 2000.
260. Sparks, M.J. et al., Pre-exercise carbohydrate ingestion: effect of the glycemic index on endurance exercise performance, *Med. Sci. Sports Exerc.*, 30:844, 1998.
261. Stannard, S.R., Constantini, N.W., and Miller J.C., The effect of glycemic index on plasma glucose and lactate levels during incremental exercise, *Int. J. Sport Nutr. Exerc. Metab.*, 10:51, 2000.

262. Wee, S. et al., Influence of high and low glycemic index meals on endurance running capacity, *Med. Sci. Sports Exerc.*, 31:393, 1999.
263. Febbraio, M.A. and Stewart, K.L., CHO feeding before prolonged exercise: effect of glycemic index on muscle glycogenolysis and exercise performance, *J. Appl. Physiol.*, 81:1115, 1996.
264. Burke, L.M. et al., Carbohydrate intake during prolonged cycling minimizes effect of glycemic index of preexercise meal, *J. Appl. Physiol.*, 85:2220, 1998.
265. Latzka, W.A. et al., Hyperhydration: tolerance and cardiovascular effects during uncompensable exercise-heat stress, *J. Appl. Physiol.*, 84:1858, 1998.
266. Lyons, T. et al., Effects of glycerol-induced hyperhydration prior to exercise in the heat on sweating and core temperature, *Med. Sci. Sports Exerc.*, 22:477, 1990.
267. Hitchens, S. et al., Glycerol hyperhydration improves cycle time trial performance in hot humid conditions, *Eur. J. Appl. Physiol.*, 80:494, 1999.
268. Montner, P. et al., Pre-exercise glycerol hydration improves cycling endurance time, *Int. J. Sports Med.*, 17:27, 1996.
269. Scheet, T.P., Webster, M.J., and Wagoner, K.D., Effectiveness of glycerol as a rehydrating agent, *Int. J. Sport Nut. Exerc. Metab.*, 11:63, 2001.
270. Hilsendager, D. and Karpovich, P.V., Ergogenic effect of glycine and niacin separately and in combination, *Res. Q.*, 35:389, 1964.
271. Miura, T. et al., Effect of guarana on exercise in normal and epinephrine-induced glycogenolytic mice, *Biol. Pharm. Bull.*, 21:646, 1998.
272. Gropper, S.S., Smith, J.L., and Groff, J.L., *Advanced Nutrition and Human Metabolism*, 4th ed., Thomson-Wadworth: Belmont, CA, 502, 2004.
273. American College of Sports Medicine, American Dietetic Association, and Dietitians of Canada, Nutrition and Athletic Performance: Joint Position Statement, *Med. Sci. Sports Exerc.*, 32:2130, 2000.
274. Barr, S.I., Effects of dehydration on exercise performance, *Can. J. Appl. Physiol.*, 24:164, 1999.
275. Brooks, G. et al., *Exercise Physiology: Human Bioenergetics and its Applications*, 3rd ed., McGraw-Hill: New York, chap 6, 2000.
276. Foster, C., Costill, D.L., and Fink, W.J., Effects of preexercise feedings on endurance performance, *Med. Sci. Sports*, 11:1, 1979.
277. McNaughton, L., Dalton, B., and Tarr, J., Inosine supplementation has no effect on aerobic or anaerobic cycling performance, *Int. J. Sport Nutr.*, 9:333, 1999.
278. Starling, R.D. et al., Effect of inosine supplementation on aerobic and anaerobic cycling performance, *Med. Sci. Sports Exerc.*, 28:1193, 1996.
279. Williams, M.H. et al., Effect of inosine supplementation on 3-mile treadmill run performance and VO_2 peak, *Med. Sci. Sports Exerc.*, 22:517, 1990.
280. Watkins, O. and Douglas, D.E., Health food supplements prepared from kelp—a source of elevated urinary arsenic, *Clin. Toxicol.*, 8:325, 1975.
281. Phinney, S.D. et al., The human metabolic response to chronic ketosis without caloric restriction: preservation of submaximal exercise capability with reduced carbohydrate oxidation, *Metabolism*, 32:769, 1983.

282. Brouns, F. et al., Chronic oral lactate supplementation does not affect lactate disappearance from blood after exercise, *Int. J. Sport Nutr.*, 5:117, 1995.

283. Bryner, R.W. et al., Effect of lactate consumption on exercise performance, *J. Sports Med. Phys. Fitness*, 38:116, 1998.

284. Swensen, T. et al., Adding polylactate to a glucose polymer solution does not improve endurance, *Int. J. Sports Med.*, 15:430, 1994.

285. Fahey, T.D. et al., The effects of ingesting polylactate or glucose polymer drinks during prolonged exercise, *Int. J. Sport Nutr.*, 1:249, 1991.

286. Pelleymounter, M.A. et al., Effects of the obese gene product on body weight regulation in ob/ob mice, *Science*, 269:540, 1995.

287. Heymsfield, S.B. et al., Recombinant leptin for weight loss in obese and lean adults: a randomized, controlled, dose-escalation trial, *JAMA*, 282:1568, 1999.

288. Layman, D.K., Role of leucine in protein metabolism during exercise and recovery, *Can. J. Appl. Physiol.*, 27:646, 2002.

289. Williams, M.H., *Nutrition for Health, Fitness & Sport*, 7th ed., McGraw-Hill: New York, 225, 2004.

290. Williams, M.H., *Nutrition for Health, Fitness & Sport*, 7th ed., McGraw-Hill: New York, 307, 2004.

291. Liu, L., Borowski, G., and Rose, L.I., Hypomagnesemia in a tennis player, *Physican Sportsmed.*, 11:79, 1983.

292. Lamb, D.R. and Brodowicz, G.R., Optimal use of fluids of varying formulations to minimise exercise-induced disturbances in homeostasis, *Sports Med.*, 3:247, 1986.

293. Beckers, E.J. et al., Gastric emptying of carbohydrate-medium chain triglyceride suspensions at rest, *Int. J. Sports Med.*, 13:581, 1992.

294. Berning, J.R., The role of medium-chain triglycerides in exercise, *Int. J. Sport Nutr.*, 6:121, 1996.

295. Bach, A.C. and Babayan, V.K., Medium-chain triglycerides: an update, *Am. J. Clin. Nutr.*, 36:950, 1982.

296. Van Zyl, C. et al., Effects of medium-chain triglyceride ingestion on fuel metabolism and cycling performance, *J. Appl. Physiol.*, 80:2217, 1996.

297. Goedecke, J.H. et al., Effects of medium-chain triacylglycerol ingested with carbohydrate on metabolism and exercise performance, *Int. J. Sport Nutr.*, 9:35, 1999.

298. Satabin, P. et al., Metabolic and hormonal responses to lipid and carbohydrate diets during exercise in man, *Med. Sci. Sports Exerc.*, 19:218, 1987.

299. Jeukendrup, A.E. et al., Effects of medium-chain triacylglycerol and carbohydrate ingestion during exercise on substrate utilization and subsequent cycling performance, *Am. J. Clin. Nutr.*, 67:397, 1998.

300. Fushiki, T.K. et al., Swimming capacity of mice is increased by chronic consumption of medium-chain triglycerides, *J. Nutr.*, 125:531, 1995.

301. Misell, L.M. et al., Chronic medium-chain triacylglycerol consumption and endurance performance in trained runners, *J. Sports Med. Phys. Fitness*, 41:210, 2001.

302. Weight, L.M. et al., Vitamin and mineral status of trained athletes including the effects of supplementation, *Am. J. Clin. Nutr.*, 47:186, 1988.

303. Weight, L.M. et al., Vitamin and mineral supplementation: effect on the running performance of trained athletes, *Am. J. Clin. Nutr.*, 47:162, 1988.

304. Bergstrom, J. et al., Effect of nicotinic acid on physical working capacity and on metabolism of muscle glycogen in man, *J. Appl. Physiol.*, 26:170, 1969.

305. Murray, R. et al., Physiological and performance responses to nicotinic-acid ingestion during exercise, *Med. Sci. Sports Exerc.*, 27:1057, 1995.

306. Pernow, B. and Saltin, B., Availability of substrates and capacity for prolonged heavy exercise in man, *J. Appl. Physiol.*, 31:416, 1971.

307. Norris, B., Schade, D.S., and Eaton, R.P., Effects of altered free fatty acid mobilization on the metabolic response to exercise, *J. Clin. Endocrinol. Metab.*, 46:254, 1978.

308. Taylor, J.C. et al., Octacosanol in human health, *Nutr.*, 19:192, 2003.

309. Raastad, T., Hostmark, A.T., and Stromme, S.B., Omega-3 fatty acid supplementation does not improve maximal aerobic power, anaerobic threshold and running performance in well-trained soccer players, *Scand. J. Med. Sci. Sports*, 7:25, 1997.

310. Oostenbrug, G.S. et al., Exercise performance, red blood cell deformability, and lipid peroxidation: effects of fish oil and vitamin E, *J. Appl. Physiol.*, 83:746, 1997.

311. Halson, S.L. et al., Immunological responses to overreaching in cyclists, *Med. Sci. Sports Exerc.*, 35:854, 2003.

312. Lehmann, M., Foster, C., and Keul, J., Overtraining in endurance athletes: a brief review, *Med. Sci. Sports Exerc.*, 25:854, 1993.

313. Antonio, J. and Stout, J.R., *Sports Supplements*, Lippincott Williams & Wilkins: Philadelphia, 284, 2001.

314. Webster, M.J., Physiological and performance responses to supplementation with thiamin and pantothenic acid derivatives, *Eur. J. Appl. Physiol.*, 77:486, 1998.

315. Nice, C. et al., The effects of panthothenic acid on human exercise capacity, *J. Sports Med.*, 24:26, 1984.

316. Cade, R., Effects of phosphate loading on 2,3-diphosphoglycerate and maximal oxygen uptake, *Med. Sci. Sports Exerc.*, 16:263, 1984.

317. Kreider, R.B. et al., Effects of phosphate loading on oxygen uptake, ventilatory anaerobic threshold, and run performance, *Med. Sci. Sports Exerc.*, 22:250, 1990.

318. Kreider, R.B. et al., Effects of phosphate loading on metabolic and myocardial responses to maximal and endurance exercise, *Int. J. Sport Nutr.*, 2:20, 1992.

319. Stewart, I. et al., Phosphate loading and the effects on VO_{2max} in trained cyclists, *Res. Q. Exerc. Sport*, 61:80, 1990.

320. Bredle, D.L. et al., Phosphate supplementation, cardiovascular function, and exercise performance in humans, *J. Appl. Physiol.*, 65:1821, 1988.

321. Duffy, D.J. and Conlee, R.K., Effects of phosphate loading on leg power and high intensity treadmill exercise, *Med. Sci. Sports Exerc.*, 18:674, 1986.

322. Lemon, P.W., Effects of exercise on dietary protein requirements, *Int. J. Sport Nutr.*, 8:426, 1998.

323. Block, G. et al., Nutrient sources in the American diet: quantitative data from the NHANES II survey: Macronutrients and fats, *Am. J. Epidemiol.*, 122:27, 1985.

324. Esmark, B. et al., Timing of postexercise protein intake is important for muscle hypertrophy with resistance training in elderly humans, *J. Physiol.*, 353:301, 2001.

325. Rasmussen, B.B. et al., An oral essential amino acid-carbohydrate supplement enhances muscle protein anabolism after resistance exercise, *J. Appl. Physiol.*, 88:386, 2000.

326. Borsheim, E. et al., Essential amino acids and muscle protein recovery from resistance exercise, *Am. J. Physiol. Endocrinol. Metab.*, 283:E648, 2002.

327. Tipton, K.D. et al., Timing of amino acid-carbohydrate ingestion alters anabolic response of muscle to resistance exercise, *Am. J. Physiol. Endocrinol. Metab.*, 281:E197, 2001.

328. Kreider, R.B., Dietary supplements and the promotion of muscle growth with resistance exercise, *Sports Med.*, 27:97, 1999.

329. Van Loon, L.J. et al., Ingestion of protein hydrolysate and amino acid-carbohydrate mixtures increases postexercise plasma insulin responses in men, *J. Nutr.*, 130:2508, 2000.

330. Jentjens, R.L. et al., Addition of protein and amino acids to carbohydrate does not enhance postexercise muscle glycogen synthesis, *J. Appl. Physiol.*, 91:839, 2001.

331. Roy, B.D. et al., Macronutrient intake and whole body protein metabolism following resistance exercise, *Med. Sci. Sports Exerc.*, 32:1412, 2000.

332. Fogt, D.L. and Ivy, J.L., Effects of postexercise carbohydrate-protein supplement on skeletal muscle glycogen storage, *Med. Sci. Sports Exerc.*, 32:S60, 2000.

333. Haub, M.D. et al., Effect of protein source on resistive-training-induced changes in body composition and muscle size in older men, *Am. J. Clin. Nutr.*, 76:511, 2002.

334. Boirie, Y. et al., Slow and fast dietary proteins differently modulate postprandial protein accretion, *Proc. Nat. Acad. Sci.*, 94:14930, 1997.

335. Dangin, M. et al., The digestion rate of protein is an independent regulating factor of postprandial protein retention, *Am. J. Physiol. Endocrinol. Metab.*, 280:E340, 2001.

336. Niles, E.S. et al., Carbohydrate-protein drink improves time to exhaustion after recovery from endurance exercise, *J. Exerc. Physiol.*, 4:45, 2001.

337. Maritim, A. et al., Effects of pycnogenol treatment on oxidative stress in streptozotocin-induced diabetic rats, *J. Biochem, Molec. Toxicol.*, 17:193, 2003.

338. Morrison, M.A, Spriet, L.L, and Dyck, D.J., Pyruvate ingestion for 7 days does not improve aerobic performance in well-trained individuals, *J. Appl. Physiol.*, 89:549, 2000.

339. Stanko, R.T. et al., Enhanced leg exercise endurance with a high-carbohydrate diet and dihydroxyacetone and pyruvate, *J. Appl. Physiol.*, 69:1651, 1990.

340. Stanko, R.T. et al., Enhancement of arm exercise endurance capacity with dihydroxyacetone and pyruvate, *J. Appl. Physiol.*, 68:119, 1990.

341. Kalman, D. et al., Effects of pyruvate supplementation on body composition and mood, *Curr. Ther. Res.*, 59:793, 1998.

342. Vukovich, M., Fat reduction. In *Sports Supplements*, Antonio, J. and Stout, J.R., Eds., Lippincott Williams & Wilkins: Philadelphia, 101, 2001.

343. Winters, L.R. et al., Riboflavin requirements and exercise adaptation in older women, *Am. J. Clin. Nutr.*, 56:526, 1992.

344. Belko, A.Z. et al., Effects of exercise on riboflavin requirements of young women, *Am. J. Clin. Nutr.*, 37:509, 1983.

345. Soares, M.J. et al., The effect of exercise on the riboflavin status of adult men, *Brit. J. Nutr.*, 69:541, 1993.

346. Haralambie, G., Vitamin B_2 status in athletes and the influence of riboflavin administration on neuromuscular irritability, *Nutr. Metab.*, 20:1, 1976.

347. Hellsten, Y., Skadhauge, L., and Bangsbo J., Effect of ribose supplementation on resynthesis of adenine nucleotides after intense intermittent training in humans, *Am. J. Physiol. Reg. Integ. Comp. Physiol.*, 286:R182, 2004.

348. Op 't Eijnde, B. et al., No effects of oral ribose supplementation on repeated maximal exercise and de novo ATP resynthesis, *J. Appl. Physiol.*, 91:2275, 2001.

349. Kreider, R.B. et al., Effects of oral D-ribose supplementation on anaerobic capacity and selected metabolic markers in healthy males, *Int. J. Sport Nutr. Exerc. Metab.*, 3:76, 2003.

350. Berardi, J.M. and Ziegenfuss, T.N., Effects of ribose supplementation on repeated sprint performance in men, *J. Strength Cond. Res.*, 17:47, 2003.

351. Poirier, L.A. et al., Blood determinations of S-adenosylmethionine, S-adenosylhomocysteine, and homocysteine, *Canc. Epidemiol. Biomarkers Prev.*, 10:649, 2001.

352. Applegate, E., Effective nutritional ergogenic aids, *Int. J. Sport Nutr.*, 8:229, 1999.

353. Verbitsky, O. et al., Effect of ingested sodium bicarbonate on muscle force, fatigue, and recovery, *J. Appl. Physiol.*, 83:333, 1997.

354. Stephens, T. et al., Effect of sodium bicarbonate on muscle metabolism during intense endurance cycling, *Med. Sci. Sports Exerc.*, 34:614, 2002.

355. Price, M., Moss, P., and Rance, S., Effects of sodium bicarbonate ingestion on prolonged intermittent exercise, *Med. Sci. Sports Exerc.*, 35:1303, 2003.

356. Matson, L. and Tran, Z., Effects of sodium bicarbonate ingestion on anaerobic performance: a meta-analytic review, *Int. J. Sport Nutr.*, 3:2, 1993.

357. Maughan, R., King, D., and Lea, T., Dietary supplements, *J. Sports Sci.*, 22:95, 2004.

358. Horswill, C.A., Effects of bicarbonate, citrate, and phosphate loading on performance, *Int. J. Sport Nutr.*, 5:S111, 1995.

359. Cox, G. and Jenkins, D.G., The physiological and ventilatory responses to repeated 60 s sprints following sodium citrate ingestion, *J. Sports Sci.*, 14:469, 1994.

360. Kowalchuk, J.M. et al., The effect of citrate loading on exercise performance, acid-base balance and metabolism, *Eur. J. Appl. Physiol.*, 58:858, 1989.

361. Parry-Billings, M. and MacLaren, D.P., The effect of sodium bicarbonate and sodium citrate ingestion on anaerobic power during intermittent exercise, *Eur. J. Appl. Physiol.*, 55:224, 1986.

362. McNaughton, L. and Cedero, R., Sodium citrate ingestion and its effects on maximal anaerobic exercise of different durations, *Eur. J. Appl. Physiol.*, 64:36, 1992.

363. Potteiger, J.A. et al., The effects of buffer ingestion on metabolic factors related to distance running performance, *Eur. J. Appl. Physiol.*, 72:365, 1996.

364. Potteiger, J.A. et al., Sodium citrate ingestion enhances 30 km cycling performance, *Int. J. Sports Med.*, 17:7, 1996.

365. Rauch, H.G. et al., Effects of ingesting a sports bar versus glucose polymer on substrate utilization and ultra-endurance performance, *Int. J. Sports Med.*, 20:252, 1999.

366. Burns, J.H. and Berning, J.R., Sports beverages. In *Macroelements, Water, and Electrolytes in Sports Nutrition*, Driskell. J.A. and Wolinsky, I., Eds., CRC Press: Boca Raton, FL, 1999.

367. Stricker, E.M. and Sved, A.F., Thirst, *Nutrition*, 16:821, 2000.

368. Passe, D.H., Horn, M., and Murray, R., The effects of beverage carbonation on sensory responses and voluntary fluid intake following exercise, *Int. J. Sport Nutr.*, 7:286, 1997.

369. Murray, R., The effects of consuming carbohydrate-electrolyte beverages on gastric emptying and fluid absorption during and following exercise, *Sports Med.*, 4:322, 1987.

370. Wemple, R.D., Morocco, T.S., and Mack, G.S., Influence of sodium replacement on fluid ingestion following exercise-induced dehydration, *Int. J. Sports Med.*, 7:104, 1997.

371. Yatabe, Y. et al., Effects of taurine administration in rat skeletal muscles on exercise, *J. Ortho. Sci.*, 8:415, 2003.

372. Matsuzaki, Y. et al., Decreased taurine concentration in skeletal muscles after exercise for various durations, *Med. Sci. Sports Exerc.*, 34:793, 2002.

373. Doyle, M.R., Webster, M.J., and Erdmann, L.D., Allithiamine ingestion does not enhance isokinetic parameters of muscle performance, *Int. J. Sport Nutr.*, 7:39, 1997.

374. Knippel, M. et al., The action of thiamin on the production of lactic acid in cyclists, *Med. Sport*, 39:11, 1986.

375. Jentjens, R.L. and Jeukendrup, A.E., Effects of pre-exercise ingestion of trehalose, galactose and glucose on subsequent metabolism and cycling performance, *Eur. J. Appl. Physiol.*, 88(4–5):459–465, 2003.

376. Antonio, J. et al., The effects of Tribulus terrestris on body composition and exercise performance in resistance-trained males, *Int. J. Sport Nutr. Exerc. Metab.*, 10:208, 2000.

377. Segura, R. and Ventura, J., Effect of L-tryptophan supplementation on exercise performance, *Int. J. Sports Med.*, 9:301, 1988.

378. Stensrud, T. et al., L-tryptophan supplementation does not improve running performance, *Int. J. Sports Med.*, 13:481, 1992.

379. Cunliffe, A., Obeid, O.A., and Powell-Tuck, J., A placebo controlled investigation of the effects of tryptophan or placebo on subjective and objective measures of fatigue, *Eur. J. Clin. Nutr.*, 52:425, 2001.

380. Struder, H.K. et al., Influence of paroxetine, branched-chain amino acids and tyrosine on neuroendocrine system responses and fatigue in humans, *Horm. Metab. Res.*, 30:188, 1998.

381. Chinevere, T.D. et al., Effects of L-tyrosine and carbohydrate ingestion on endurance exercise performance, *J. Appl. Physiol.*, 93:1590, 2002.

382. Jentjens, R.L. and Jeukendrup, A.E., Effect of acute and short-term administration of vanadyl sulphate on insulin sensitivity in healthy active humans, *Int. J. Sport Nutr. Exerc. Metab.*, 12:470, 2002.

383. Fawcett, J.P. et al., The effect of oral vanadyl sulfate on body composition and performance in weight-training athletes, *Int. J. Sport Nutr.*, 6:382, 1996.

384. Bereczki, D. and Fekete, I., A systematic review of vinpocetine therapy in acute ischaemic stroke, *Eur. J. Clin. Pharmacol.*, 55:349, 1999.

385. Paulo, T. et al., [3H]Noradrenaline-releasing action of vinpocetine in the isolated main pulmonary artery of the rabbit, *J. Pharm. Pharmacol.*, 38:668, 1986.

386. Wald, G., Brouha, L., and Johnson, R., Experimental human vitamin A deficiency and ability to perform muscular exercise, *Am. J. Physiol.*, 137:551, 1942.

387. Manore, M.M. and Leklem, J.E., Effect of carbohydrate and vitamin B_6 on fuel substrates during exercise in women, *Med. Sci. Sports Exerc.*, 20:233, 1988.

388. Schaumburg. H. et al., Sensory neuropathy from pyridoxine abuse. A new megavitamin syndrome, *New Eng. J. Med.*, 309:445, 1983.

389. Tin-May-Than et al., The effect of vitamin B_{12} on physical performance capacity, *Br. J. Nutr.*, 40:269, 1978.

390. Bucci, L., *Nutrients as Ergogenic Aids for Sports and Exercise*, CRC Press: Boca Raton, FL, chap. 3, 1993.

391. Shephard, R.J., Vitamin E and athletic performance, *J. Sports Med. Phys. Fitness*, 23:461, 1983.

392. Smolak, L., Murnen, S.K., and Ruble, A.E., Female athletes and eating problems: a meta-analysis, *Int. J. Eating Dis.*, 27:371, 2000.

393. Jakicic, J.M. et al., American College of Sports Medicine position stand: appropriate intervention strategies for weight loss and prevention of weight regain for adults, *Med. Sci. Sports Exerc.*, 33:2145, 2001.

394. Richelsen, B. et al., Regional differences in triglyceride breakdown in human adipose tissue: effects of catecholamines, insulin, and prostaglandin E2, *Metabolism*, 40:990, 1991.

395. Galitzky, J. et al., Alpha 2-antagonist compounds and lipid mobilization: evidence for a lipid mobilizing effect of oral yohimbine in healthy male volunteers, *Eur. J. Clin. Invest.*, 18:587, 1988.

396. Tam, S.W., Worcel, M., and Wyllie, M., Yohimbine: a clinical review, *Pharmacol. Ther.*, 91:215, 2001.

397. Krotkiewski, M. et al., Zinc and muscle strength and endurance, *Acta Physiol. Scand.*, 116:309, 1982.

Printed and bound by CPI Group (UK) Ltd, Croydon, CR0 4YY

23/10/2024

01778239-0007